Helping and Healing

Helping and Healing
Religious Commitment in Health Care

EDMUND D. PELLEGRINO
DAVID C. THOMASMA

WITH THE EDITORIAL ASSISTANCE OF
David G. Miller

GEORGETOWN UNIVERSITY PRESS / WASHINGTON, D.C.

Georgetown University Press, Washington, D.C.   20007
© 1997 by Georgetown University Press. All rights reserved.
Printed in the United States of America.
10   9   8   7   6   5   4   3   2   1   1997
THIS VOLUME IS PRINTED ON ACID-FREE OFFSET BOOKPAPER.

Library of Congress Cataloging-in-Publication Data

Pellegrino, Edmund D.,   1920–
    [Medicina per vocazione.   English]
    Helping and healing   :   religious commitment in health care /
Edmund D. Pellegrino, David C. Thomasma.
          p.   cm.
    Translated from Italian.
    Includes bibliographical references.
    1. Medical ethics.   2. Christian ethics.   I. Thomasma, David
C., 1939–   . II. Title.
R725.56.P45513   1997
174'.2—dc21
ISBN 0-87840-643-3 (pbk)

                                                      96-46598

Contents

116523

Acknowledgments

We would like to acknowledge the help of Doris Thomasma and Marti Patchell in typing various parts of this manuscript into our computers and, along with Karin Dean, making the arrangements whereby we were able to finish the manuscript with the least disruptions to our schedule. David Miller, as always, assisted us in final copyediting and checking the references. We are grateful for his constant help. Clementine Pellegrino was often a gracious hostess, enabling us to work in a comfortable home environment as well. Her support is deeply appreciated. Joan Allman also earned our gratitude for initially typing a substantial number of chapters in WordPerfect. This work was supported by the Office of Research at Loyola University of Chicago, whose Director, Thomas Bennett, Ph.D., aided us more than once. We want to thank him, too. Finally we are grateful to Professor Erich Loewy, M.D., for his thorough and helpful comments on an earlier draft of this book. He has prompted us to develop more fully those points at which skeptics, secular humanists, and religious believers may come together in their shared commitment to the healing of the sick. He has also helped us to delineate more clearly the relationship between reason and faith.

An Italian translation of this book appeared as *Medicina per vocazione: Impegno religioso in medicina*, trans. Fr. Antonio Puca (Rome: Editiones Dehoniane, 1994). Portions of this book were taken from previously published articles:

Edmund D. Pellegrino, "The Trials of Job: A Physician's Meditation," *Linacre Quarterly* 56, no. 2 (1989): 76–88; "The Caring Ethic: The Relationship of Physician to Patient," in *Caring, Curing, Coping: Nursing-Physician Relationships*, ed. Anne H. Bishop and John R. Scudder, Jr. (Alabama: University of Alabama Press, 1985) pp. 8–30; "Agape and Ethics: Some Reflections on Medical Morals from a Catholic Christian Perspective," in *Catholic Perspectives on Medical Morals*, ed. Edmund D. Pellegrino, John P. Langan, and John C. Harvey (Dordrecht, Holland and Boston, Mass.: Kluwer, 1989), pp. 277–300; "Health Care: A Vocation to Justice and Love," in *The Professions in*

Ethical Context: Vocations to Justice (Proceedings of the Theology Institute of Villanova University), ed. Francis A. Eigo (Villanova, Pennsylvania: Villanova University Press, 1986), pp. 97–126.

David C. Thomasma, "Moral Integrity and Healthcare Leadership," *Healthcare Executive* 8, no. 1 (1993): 29; "Healthcare Management and Ethics: Access to Healthcare," *Healthcare Executive* 7, no. 2 (1992): 30; "The Ethics of Caring for Vulnerable Individuals," in American Speech-Language-Hearing Association, *Reflections on Ethics* (Washington, D.C.: American Speech-Language-Hearing Association, 1990), pp. 39–45.

Introduction

Our previous books have attempted to set forth the beginnings of a philosophically grounded moral philosophy for medicine.[1] The present book represents a further step in our endeavor to develop a more complete account of such a moral philosophy. In this book we try to encompass the religious sources of medical morality. In doing so, we acknowledge our personal commitment to a view in which moral philosophy and theology are mutually reinforcing endeavors. This religious tradition recognizes a place for human reason within faith, but also subscribes to the need for human reason to be illumined by the authoritative word of Scripture and tradition. We take a middle course between the straightforward fideism of fundamentalists, on the one hand, and the reductions of moral philosophy to moral neutralism, relativism, or sociobiological determinism, on the other.

Our hope is to steer a clear path between excessive mistrust and undue exaltation of human reason. Religious faith has sometimes taken on the quality of a passionate prejudice or a retreat into comfortable cliches and prefabricated answers. These aberrations do not illuminate the problem of suffering and healing in any useful way. On the other hand, an outright secular humanism seems seriously antiquated in a postnuclear age. The notion that human nature and human society are good and perfectible, an inheritance from the Enlightenment, seems to many, in light of the massive technological and political cruelties of the twentieth century, to be the unkindest belief of all. As contemporary rabbis remind us, one cannot do moral philosophy and theology today without taking the Holocaust into account.

We approach moral philosophy in the spirit of Aristotle and Aquinas. Thus we acknowledge the strengths and weaknesses of human reason in the theoretical and practical sciences. From this perspective we propose to examine how religious commitments shape our perceptions about health care and medicine as well as the moral choices that must be made in the care of sick persons. What influence, we will ask, does religion have on the kind of person the health professional should be, on the health care policies a nation should adopt, and on what constitutes healing in the fullest sense of that term? Our whole enterprise is an attempt to grasp the Christian message as it engages the world of the sick—daily, personally, and in concrete situations. What we seek is an augmentation of philosophic ethics by Christian insights into the meaning and purpose of human life.[2]

This attempt must struggle with the apparent clash between reason and faith. A belief in the powers of reason prompts us to ask the questions posed in this text. It also functions as a check on uncritical fideism. Religious faith modulates and influences the kinds of questions we raise. Reason is needed to divest oneself of any monochromatic position uncritically accepted. When two persons are inspired by their faith and cannot agree, reason can function to close the gap between them. Reason explores their common ground: the nature of human life, suffering, and the community.[3] Yet reason itself needs to be checked from another perspective. The fallibility of human reason is too well established to expect perfection in the way it comprehends so rich a tapestry as human life, especially when so many threads in that tapestry are intuitive, emotive, and experiential.

With full recognition of the difficulties, our effort is to fashion a "Christian philosophy" of medicine, an amalgam of reason inspired by faith.[4] We do not propose to construct a moral theology of medicine, although some of what we offer would be consistent with such an enterprise.[5] Rather we are concerned with the kinds of responses religious people are called upon to make to the multitudinous and complex dilemmas of today's medical practice and medical ethics.

CRUCIAL DEFINITIONS

It is important, therefore, to define "religion," "theology," and "religious perspective" as we use them in this text. They are distinct from one another and not synonymous.

"Religion" we take to be any set of beliefs that involve at the outset a commitment of faith. This commitment of faith functions as an initial starting point for thinking and acting. Every statement of fact, every pronouncement about the world, starts from a belief about the world and about our perception of it. What makes religious belief different is that it accepts a source of reality and morality outside, beyond, and sometimes over and against human beings, in the sense of a check on humanity's instincts and actions. In our understanding, then, religion may or may not involve ritual and liturgy. Humanists who call upon a conglomerate of the best of human thought, or of humanity as an ideal "Humanity," would fall under this definition of religion. Their commitment of faith is to the more admirable qualities of human nature. The varieties of religious experience are many and diverse—from cosmic religion to belief in a personal saving God.[6]

When we use the phrase "religious perspective" in ethics, we mean a stance, a viewing point, a set of presuppositions about right and wrong that involves religious faith. Persons commit themselves to a particular perspective. It shapes their judgments about right and wrong and thereby, directly or indirectly, influences the major decisions of their lives. Our perspective is Christian and Roman Catholic. This perspective influences our insights about modern medicine. Many fundamental insights are shared with other Christian denominations; and a few others, with all religions. This is especially true of the fundamental themes of illness and healing discussed in our book.

Our goal is to demonstrate the possibilities of enriching and broadening the ethical enterprise in medicine by a religious perspective. This book is therefore not an exposition of Catholic thought about healing, which Pope John Paul II has so eloquently adumbrated in his writings.[7] This is not an apologia for any religion. Rather our aim is to "mine" religions, broadly conceived, for insights that might reveal a better understanding of modern medicine and medical practice.

"Theology" we take more formally to mean an organized, systematic, and critical reflection on revealed sources of truth reflected in a faith community's history, documents, traditions, and church teachings. Broadly speaking, theology is any systematic reflection on the content of religious belief. Clearly our book is not a theological treatise.

Given these definitions, one will not find in our book a manual of medical moral theology, a summary of official teachings of Christian churches, or even a thorough exploration of topics that feature prominently in studies of theological and religious ethics, such as abortion, euthanasia, artificial insemination, reproductive issues such as in vitro fertilization, withholding and withdrawal of fluids and nutrition, brain death, and similar topics.[8] These topics are omitted, not because we believe them to be unimportant but because we wish to concentrate on a less well explored area, the ways a religious perspective shapes the central act of medicine—the healing relationship—and the ethics of that relationship.

Not all Christians will agree with either the method or the content of our perspective. Nor do we expect them to do so. Rather we want to show how someone with a religious perspective as we have defined it might approach some of the many problems in medical ethics today, and how that perspective might also shed light on the deeper questions of the theory of medicine upon which medical ethics is ultimately grounded. We also hope to show how the religious perspective differs from, supplements, and complements the dominant analytical mode of doing medical ethics.[9] Our hope is to examine the common ground for all who take a religious standpoint on biomedical ethical questions. The entire effort of any legitimate religion is to call forth the best qualities in human beings. As Richard McCormick succinctly puts it: "The Church is in the health care apostolate because it is a most concrete and effective way of communicating to human beings their real worth."[10]

We do not think this is the place to argue the rational or spiritual supremacy of one religious persuasion over another. Nonetheless our responses occur within a framework we think is consistent with our own tradition. We wish to show that religion as a source for medical morality and medical theory cannot be ignored, even in a morally heterogeneous society. To ignore religion is to ignore the oldest, most universal, and most powerful ethical force motivating human moral behavior, even today.

A BETRAYAL OF THE PROMISE OF MEDICINE

A major dilemma for our times is the clash between the values of technology and the values of medicine. Even though few people would reject modern medical advances, the use of these advances must be governed and constrained by human and moral ends.[11] In fact, the very enunciation of needs that lead to medical advances is based on moral concerns that precede the moral problems that later arise from technological advances themselves.[12]

Human and moral ends are yet to be fully identified, especially in medicine. Without them we are "abandoned" to a plethora of means and a poverty of ends. Our technology has outstripped our traditional ethical systems of thought. Small wonder that the doctor in Franz

Kafka's *Das Landartz* yells out at the end of a story about his frustrations in trying to heal, "*Betrogen!*"—that is, "Betrayed!"[13]

Like the country doctor in Kafka's story, many physicians feel betrayed by their own discipline because it has helped them control disease but ironically has also separated them from the dramatic human sufferings of their patients. Years of serious intellectual work on this problem still lie ahead, despite the growth of medical ethics and of the philosophy of medicine. When Martin Heidegger was asked to summarize his years of effort exploring the relation of person and technology and the promise of the future, he opined: "Only a God can save us."[14] He could not formulate a philosophical answer. This is a cop-out. What is needed is not a God who might rescue us from our own inventions. Rather what is needed is nothing less than a rational ethic for human beings in a technological era.[15]

The problem is far too complex to fix blame, especially to castigate medical education and the health care delivery system. The reason is that ends are difficult to articulate and, once reached, are most likely to function as means to other as yet unarticulated ends. This is why John Dewey called ends "ends-in-view."[16] A very complex set of values governs the care of individuals and groups in our society. And medicine is in the thick of this effort. Medical progress puts medicine squarely into confrontation with themes of human life, the duties of society toward human beings, and the moral status of scientific research. The treatment of the ill requires sensitivity to patient values, and care for persons rather than for political and economic abstractions. Medical decisions must fuse the good of the patient with scientifically correct decisions. Thus, medicine invariably turns on a moral option—as a fusion of technology and morality in which the regulating element is what ought to be done, not only what can be done.

In this book, we hold up a mirror of self-examination to an ancient profession. We focus especially on the religious dimension of health and healing, and its callings to both patients and professionals. Being sick and being healed mean that, in the end, we can demand nothing less than competent and compassionate, scientific and learned physicians intensely aware that their patients and they themselves share the perplexities of the human condition.

A major part of that condition is the effort of constant, ongoing reflection on the values that govern health care interactions. This leads to intensified interest in biomedical ethics. It also reveals that the vision behind our ethical stances on specific issues is a religious one, though this is seldom acknowledged as such.

SECULAR AND RELIGIOUS PERSPECTIVES

Today's energetic expansion of interest in biomedical ethics has taken place in a predominately secular and therefore necessarily morally pluralistic society. To deal with pluralism, medical ethics has been largely analytical, procedural, and consensual in approach. Indeed, with this approach accord is being reached on a variety of vital ethical issues, e.g., widespread acceptance of informed consent in everyday medical practice as well as in research medicine, growth of respect for the autonomy of the person, and the various recommendations of the President's Commission and other bodies. [17]

Successful as the current approach has been, it neglects one of the most pervasive and significant sources of morality—namely, religious commitment. The reality is that for many people—health professionals, patients, laypersons, policy makers—religion is still accepted as the ultimate source of morality. The majority of humans still acknowledge a reality beyond the human that serves as a source for defining what is right and good and what kind of person one ought to be. While the content of the morality derived from a transcendental source may vary, most people rely on such a source as their justification of last resort when challenged to explain why they made one moral choice rather than another.

The reality of religious influences cannot be entirely submerged. If it is, ethical discourse might remain superficial or, at best, neglectful of an important moral dimension. If it is denied, we cannot grapple with one of the most powerful and restorative forces in medical care. Further, if religious influence is denied, insights about the deeper meanings of illness and healing in a community of healers may also be missed. True moral accord becomes difficult, and discord persists despite surface agreement on procedure and protocol in making moral decisions. Thus the illusion of accord takes precedence over the reality. [18] Ethical procedure supersedes moral substance, and the necessary engagement with fundamental issues is postponed.

But engagement with the deeper foundations of biomedical ethics can no longer be postponed. Ethics is more than the application of prima facie principles to specific cases. It is also an invitation to a way of life, to the complete formation of the human person. In medicine, ethics not only resolves dilemmas; it also has the positive function of so ordering the process of healing and decision making as to enhance the humanity of the sick person and of the health worker as well. Without taking religious commitments and realities into account, these larger positive functions of medical ethics cannot be satisfactorily fulfilled.

The problems are universal. Insights about these problems in one tradition often have parallels in other religious traditions. Thus this book is addressed to all who acknowledge the importance of philosophical medical ethics but whose religious commitment convinces them of the need for a fuller response than philosophical ethical stances to the challenges in today's scientific, technological, and cultural revolutions. This book has applicability for secular professionals as well. If they are conscientious about respecting the personhood and values of their patients, they too must take into account their patients' religious values. We hope they will find herein an appreciation for the religious dimension of medicine and its ethics in the lives of a great number of their patients. Without respecting this dimension they cannot fulfill their obligation to act in the patient's best interests.

Our concern therefore goes beyond the formalism that characterizes contemporary medical ethics. In making this assertion we realize that we open up a very old and still very vexed question—the apparent conflicts that may occur between a philosophically based ethic that acknowledges only human reason and one that draws on religious belief and seeks its inspiration from a faith commitment. As Robert Sokolowski notes:

> "Christian faith is said to be in accordance with reason and yet to go beyond reason. This claim immediately gives rise to a difficulty. On the one hand the concordance of faith with reason seems to reduce Christian belief to rational thinking and to natural human experience; on the other hand the difference between faith and reason seems to make belief unreasonable and arbitrary."[19]

What happens when an individual's reason tells her that what she holds in faith to be "true" does not appear to be so, or wars against experience? Her religion might teach that euthanasia is wrong, and yet she might find abhorrent the terminal sufferings of a patient with cancer of the head and neck and on some days think that active euthanasia might be appropriate. Or individuals contemplating the beauty of nature might feel insignificant in the billions of years that shaped our planet and be tempted to rethink their commitment to the doctrines of creation, redemption, and salvation to which they previously adhered. If the beliefs are challenged too much by reason, a ready answer always at hand is that such beliefs are ultimately "mysteries" and not subject to reason but, rather, to the assent that comes from a gift of faith from God. Further, given the wounded state of human nature (something that secularists deny but for which there seems to be a great deal of evidence), those who believe are asked to trust not in "fallen" human nature but in God. The mysteries will someday be revealed to be in accord with reason but are not grasped this way at this time.

Those who trust more in human reason and remain skeptical of religious faith also believe in mysteries. *Omnia exeunt in mysterium,* all things eventually end in mystery. The nonbeliever is in no way more "rational" than the believer. The difference lies in the context of the act of belief. While a religious person believes in an outside source of truth, a nonbeliever (in our view a misnomer) makes an act of faith in his or her own mind. He or she refuses to believe in anything that does not convince as judged by the usual standards of evidence. This is just as foundational an act of faith as that employed by the religious believer, whose faith is placed in some transcendental truth.

What is common to both perspectives is one of the things we seek to dig out in this book. Every line of argument in the range of reason must start with some prelogical assumptions about the world, some act of faith, some irreducible belief.[20] These may be a belief in God, the cosmos, reason itself, Humanity, Baal, or what have you. People differ within and without religious communities about what presuppositions ought to count for carrying on moral discourse. To affirm and to deny are both "religious" acts, as we have defined them. Both actions are a response to a transcendent element in human experience—to affirm or deny it is a first act of the intellect.

So our hope is that even secular humanists will remain open to the reality of this dimension and find insights that might help them, as providers or as potential patients, to better understand and practice the art of healing.

IGNORING FUNDAMENTAL VALUES

Many health professionals today feel frustrated by the isolation of their religious beliefs from their professional practices. Too often they take this isolation for granted in a secular and pluralistic society. They feel compelled to "bracket" their deepest commitments. Yet they know also that such a compartmentalization is neither rational nor consistent with their religious beliefs. Serious illness is too clearly a challenge in the spiritual order, too directly a confrontation with the fundamental questions about the meaning of human existence. Conscientious physicians and nurses know they cannot heal truly without taking this dimension into account.

This book is an encouragement and reinforcement for those health professionals who seek to be healers in the fullest sense and also to be healed in their own lives. We also hope to encourage institutions with an explicit religious commitment to reflect critically on that commitment and to preserve it. Too many institutions under religious auspices are making dangerous moral compromises in a climate increasingly inimical to religious values. It is essential to avoid these compromises when confronting the issues of abortion, use of fetal tissue, embryo research, genetic manipulation, voluntary direct euthanasia, and involuntary direct euthanasia. These have been, are, or will be subjects of legislation. And those with religious convictions must stand firm in their conviction, and not compromise them by erecting a wall between professional life and religious commitments.

Much of the moral desuetude into which we believe the professions—medicine, law, even the ministry—have fallen is the consequence of ethical claims without a moral philosophy on which to ground them. Without a moral philosophy of medicine and an accompanying moral theology, the compass points by which policies, laws, regulations, and contracts are to be judged are lacking. Moral arguments based on utility, cost-benefit analysis, contract law, economic restraints, unbridled individualism, or the exaltation of society's needs over those of the individual are all symptoms of "moral malaise." One obvious result is the increasing willingness of some societies to depreciate the value of the most vulnerable among us: the aged, the very young, the poor, and the disenfranchised. Without the constraints of a moral philosophy that goes beyond quandary solving, claims and counterclaims compete with one another and conflict is resolved by yielding to the most energetic and strident voice.

Indeed, much of the disappointment of the professionals with their daily work derives from confusion about its moral purpose and how to resolve the challenges it poses to personal beliefs. Burnout is not just the result of physical or emotional stress. Rather its roots lie in living a lie. The steady decline of the sense of obligation—which reduces medical beneficence to simple nonmaleficence and contract fulfillment—is morally corrosive. What was once considered a duty, e.g., to efface self-interest for the sake of a patient's needs, is now considered supererogation. Patients can no longer rely on such a commitment. Many physicians grapple with the hardest struggle of all in caring for patients: constructing a synthesis between personal morality and communal expectations, especially for cutting costs in health care. Further, the growing dominance and even legitimation of physician self-interest may be the most disquieting ethical phenomenon of our times.

Most persons with religious beliefs seek sources of inspiration and aspiration beyond the minimalist tendencies of contemporary medical morality. They must be, of course, acquainted with medical ethics as a problem-solving skill, but they must also recognize its limitations. Those who profess a religion have duties over and above those prescribed by a particular system of medical ethics. A fully coherent moral philosophy is one that is open to the religious dimension as well. Our hope is that health professionals who read this book will be moved to reflect on their own religious convictions, those of their patients, the institutions in which they work, and the societies in which they reside. If our readers feel refreshed and reinforced in their religious commitment and make it integral to their professional lives, our purposes will have been fulfilled. For those without such a commitment we strive for a better appreciation of the importance of religion in the lives of their patients and their colleagues and in society at large.

NOTES

1. Edmund D. Pellegrino and David C. Thomasma, *A Philosophical Basis of Medical Practice* (New York: Oxford University Press, 1981); *For the Patient's Good: The Restoration of Beneficence in Health Care* (New York: Oxford University Press, 1988).

2. cf. Richard A. McCormick, *Health and Medicine in the Catholic Tradition* (New York: Crossroad, 1987).

3. Erich Loewy, *Suffering and the Beneficent Community* (Albany: State University of New York Press, 1991).

4. The problem of whether there is a specific "Christian philosophy" was a major part of the debates in the time of Jacques Maritain. We think there is a specific discipline, represented by this book, of religious reflection on the discipline of medicine. It is philosophical. But it is also infused by one's faith in the deeper vision that underlies many of our moral activities. As Richard Westley, *What a Modern Catholic Believes about the Right to Life* (Chicago: Thomas More, 1973), pp. 73–103, remarks of the "right to life" debate: "Catholics are the ones usually singled out by their opponents as having nonrational (religious) elements hidden behind their arguments. For some strange reason, the Catholics vehemently deny this charge, as if to match the quality of their opponents' argument which is supposedly purely rational. If that were the case, then we should expect their arguments to be conclusive. But they are not conclusive either . . . all the arguments in the debate rest on other than rational grounds; it is just that everyone seems afraid to admit it."

5. The basis of such a project has been well examined from an ecumenical standpoint in the series entitled Health, Medicine, and the Faith Traditions, developed by the Park Ridge Center, now in Chicago, Illinois. These works are published by Crossroad Press.

6. William James, *The Varieties of Religious Experience* (New York: Penguin Books, 1982); Jean Danielou, *God and the Ways of Knowing* (New York: Meridian, 1957).

7. Pope John Paul II, *Salvifici Doloris* (Washington, D.C.: United States Catholic Conference, 1984).

8. Instead, we will focus on broader themes that are now being addressed at the intersection of medicine and religion. For example, see Richard Gula, "Moral Principles Shaping Public Policy on Euthanasia"; Brendan P. Minogue, "The Exclusion of Theology from Public Policy"; Richard B. Gunderman, "Medicine and the Question of Suffering," *Second Opinion* 14 (July 1990): 72–83, 84–93, and 14–25 respectively; and Douglas Anderson, "The Physician's Experience: Witnessing Numinous Reality," *Second Opinion* 13 (March 1990): 110–123.

9. Today criticism of formalism in medical ethics has led to a critique of what is called the "Georgetown mantra," repeating the importance of the principles of autonomy, beneficence, and justice in modern health care.

10. McCormick, *Health and Medicine*, p. 20.

11. David C. Thomasma, *Human Life in the Balance* (New York: Continuum, 1990).

12. James P. Carse, "The Social Effect of Changing Attitudes towards Death," *Annals of the New York Academy of Science* 315 (November 17, 1978): 322–328.

13. Franz Kafka, *Das Landartz (The Country Doctor)*, in *The Complete Stories*, ed. Nahum N. Glatzer (New York: Schocken Books, 1971).

14. Martin Heidegger, *Discourse on Thinking* (New York: Harper and Row, 1966).

15. Thomasma, *Human Life in the Balance.*

16. John Dewey, "Means and Consequences—How, When, and What For?" in *John Dewey and Arthur F. Bentley: A Philosophical Correspondence, 1932–1951,* ed. Sidney Ratner and Jules Altman (New Brunswick, N.J.: Rutgers University Press, 1964).

17. President's Commission for the Study of Ethical Problems in Medicine and Biomedical and Behavioral Research, *Deciding to Forego Life-Sustaining Treatment: Ethical, Medical, and Legal Issues in Treatment Decisions* (Washington, D.C.: United States Government Printing Office, 1983).

18. Alasdair MacIntyre, *After Virtue* (Notre Dame, Ind.: University of Notre Dame Press, 1981).

19. Robert Sokolowski, *The God of Faith and Reason: Foundations of Christian Theology* (Notre Dame, Ind.: University of Notre Dame Press, 1982), p. xi.

20. Jacques Maritain, *The Range of Reason* (New York: Scribner's, 1952).

1

Health and Illness

Thus we love our neighbor in bringing help to his bodily needs, for our soul bears in itself seed, by reason of the likeness (between our neighbor and ourself), so that from our infirmity pity moves us to bring aid to the poverty of those in need, helping them as we would wish help given us if we were in the same great need. . . .

Augustine, *Confessions,*
trans. F. J. Sheed (Indianapolis and Cambridge:
Hackett Publishing Company, 1943), Bk. 13, Ch. 17, p. 269.

From a purely naturalistic perspective, health and illness are gains or losses in the biological lottery we call life. They are without ultimate meanings. The pain and suffering they engender are unmitigated tragedies. There is no "redemptive" aspect to suffering. In this view there can be no meaning to even a moment's suffering. Indeed, so powerful is the seeming absurdity of illness, and death, that for many it is the most powerful argument against the existence of a good God.[1] For others, the suffering and death of loved ones may be an occasion to abandon a previous faith commitment.

Here is perhaps one of the most specific areas in health care ethics in which a religious perspective counts for a difference. A providential interpretation of human existence requires that God is mindful of us: "O Lord, You have probed me, and You know me," begins Psalm 139. Each person is individually loved and tended for. God is seen as a shepherd who leads his sheep, carefully and lovingly, so that they are not harmed. Individual persons have value because salvation is an opportunity and possibility. Nothing can happen to us that has not been foreseen and has not been permitted (Matt 10:30; Luke 12:7). Faith compels the believer to affirm God's existence as an existence that matters to human beings and to the universe itself.[2] This affirmation must be made in faith when it appears to human eyes, by every natural criterion we can muster, that it is otherwise. That is why Kierkegaard called it the "leap of faith," a leap across a chasm of doubt and emptiness.[3]

SOURCE OF MEANING

A religious perspective is a source of meaning for illness and death. Illness and dying need not always be seen as useless, meaningless, and ultimately disabling. It is easy to succumb to the point of view (from a philosophical perspective) that illness is always an impairment.[4] Eric Cassell, in arguing that the proper goal of medicine is the reconstruction of the autonomy of persons, assumes this view.[5] Indeed, almost every philosopher of medicine does so.[6] If medicine attends only to the aspect of impairment (as it tends to in interventionist settings), then it misses the real challenge of enablement, empowerment, and atonement. These latter are full-blown examples of a religious dimension that is normally neglected in models of healing.

Illness can be seen as an enablement; it may enable one to grow spiritually and emotionally. It teaches finitude and appreciation for the smallest thing. A patient, taking a first meal after abdominal surgery, may never have appreciated previously how wonderful a cracker tastes! Illness can present to patients the ancient and perduring themes of reconciliation, atonement, and setting an example of courage and tenacity for others. A spinal-cord injury patient may find that nothing could give more meaning to his life than showing his son how a person confronts the losses paralysis entails. Illness can be an occasion for drawing a family together, to sacrifice for the good of another member.

As empowerment, illness can be an invitation to selflessness, calling individuals to imitate Christ or some other religious leader in their devotion to the building up of the community. Although sickness happens only to an individual, it happens in a community that stipulates the appropriate behaviors for seeking help for the illness. Thus illness can provide an opportunity for the community to demonstrate how deeply it cares. For others, it can inspire good works in the community. Some people conclude after a serious illness that God still has work for them to do and that there is so little time. In this way, disease can awaken our deepest experience of belonging to one another. If the transaction between healers and the patient is conducted with compassion and respect, the relationship itself will point to this belongingness.

Furthermore, a religious perspective helps persons deal with the inevitable question: "Why me?" Everyone facing a serious illness or accident asks this question. Atonement is one answer. Atonement in the religious sense has little to do with "making up for." Rather atonement should be taken as "at-one-ment," an effort to unite with all persons through being forgiven. This is the meaning of the Jewish feast of Yom Kippur, to apologize to all one has harmed before assembling to pray in the synagogue. Thus, one cannot go out and destroy other human beings and then pretend to be at one with them by assembling for prayer. Atonement in this meaning is also the source of the Christian ritual, in the Eucharist, of begging forgiveness before sharing the "table of the Lord." The experience of being one with other human beings can also emerge within the context of a serious illness.

One medical student, who was about to endure a very serious operation for a tumor in the spine, recalls being told by attending physicians and fellow third-year students that the experience would make her a better person and a more compassionate doctor. Her feelings were angry instead. Her "Why me?" question transformed into "Why not some other students, who could certainly profit from this lesson more than I, who am already compassionate?"

There is no final answer to questions like these, but this student decided that the lesson of illness for her was a form of atonement for not being as compassionate as she might have been in the past. Belonging to the community in a more profound way also emerges as the "lesson" of illness. A person who, prior to an accident, might have been indifferent to the problems of the disabled, after being temporarily in a wheelchair from a broken leg, might now more fully appreciate the plight of such people in society.

BECOMING ILL OR DISABLED

What is the meaning of being ill? Most people regard themselves as being in a state of health. A state of health cannot be determined absolutely. Despite all the recent attempts to define health, no better functional definition of health has been given than by Galen, who defined health as that state in which we feel able to do the things that we wish to do with a minimum of pain and discomfort.[7] This means that one can feel in a state of health, and not feel ill, even while one may have disease. Indeed, many of us have disease within us and yet are able to do the things we want to do with a minimum of discomfort and disability. Judging our own health and illness is quite subjective. It varies from person to person. One person may have absolutely nothing wrong with him, may have been checked over and over for days in a medical center, and still feel and look sick. Another may have just learned that she has Hodgkin's disease and be overjoyed after fearing that she had a less responsive form of cancer. The former is doing well but feeling worse; the latter is doing worse but feeling well.

From this relative state of balance, something happens that shakes us out of that feeling of being in a healthy state and prompts us to seek help. That balance is upset by some symptom: a pain in the chest, the finding of a lump, the loss of appetite, morning nausea, dizziness on bending over. When these symptoms are perceived as a change in the function of our whole organism, they become sufficient to lead us to seek help. We become patients when we need help in bearing a problem, a pain, a concern, an anxiety. Actually, it makes no difference whether the problem is emotional or physical; when we seek professional help, we become patients. In becoming patients we enter a new existential state of dependency and vulnerability. In this state of vulnerability called illness, the body becomes the center of our concern because it is an impediment to, rather than a willing instrument for, the things we want to do. The self dissolves into an ego and a body.[8] The task of healing is a response to this dissolution.

Another way of emphasizing this is to consider, as Eric Cassell cautions, that a sick person is not merely "a well person with the knapsack of illness strapped to his back" but a newly constituted human entity in need. One of the main functions of healing this dissolution of the person into the ego and body, then, is to reconstitute the patient's autonomy.[9]

JOB AS METAPHOR

The Book of Job is a wonderful source for a phenomenological structure of illness seen from a religious perspective. The book itself might have been a play performed around the campfire to test the theories of the Wisdom literature school of theology at the time.[10] These theories concentrated on the view that illness and bad fortune were a punishment from God.[11] As we shall see in chapter 3, this view predominates in most of the Western tradition until the present era. It is still present in the views of many about AIDS victims, for example. Job struggles against this causative view of evil in the world.

Job confronts the enigma of human suffering directly, poignantly, and in sublime poetic language. It leaves us deeply disquieted, but never indifferent. Job has been read in a multitude of ways: as a paradigm of patience; a test of righteousness; a proof that good may come from evil; an evidence of the meaninglessness of human existence; a proof of God's indifference to human suffering or of the moral ambivalence of illness. Some conclude that the answer to Job's questions is abandonment to God's will; others say that the rejection of God as a cosmic sadist is the point of the text; still others argue that human, not divine, love is the only reality we can rely upon. Whatever the interpretation, all ages have recognized that the Book of Job describes an inescapable human experience, one that each of us ultimately must confront and to which each must fashion a personal response.[12]

Job was, most of all, so beset by the unreasonableness of his own illness, and of the apparent punishment, that he dared to challenge God. He constantly protested his own innocence. This protest bordered on blasphemy. He demanded to know why he had been singled out for punishment even though he was faithful. He had played by all the rules, and now he sat on a dungheap (perhaps as a cure recommended by the physicians of his time). He felt that he had every right to expect that God would treat him with special solicitude. Was he not God's friend, faithful servant? Did he not have a right to be treated less harshly?

This is the same stream of thought that other believers, down through history, have experienced when serious illness upsets that precarious balance we call "health." What are the components of illness behavior in Job?

1) Health. Job starts out "healthy." He interprets being healthy as being prosperous, a righteous desert chieftan in the land of Uz, loved by his family, friends, and God. A contemporary surgeon or businessperson might have the same feelings of prominence in society, of having "made it," of being an integral force in society, of contributing and being rewarded for those contributions.

2) External Losses. The healthy, balanced state goes awry. Losses occur in the business. Job loses his flocks. Later his home is destroyed. All his children are killed. This is a major calamity, since the Jews and

other agrarians identified the blessings of God with their own progeny. In a profound way, external losses contribute to suffering and eventually to illness. People today are stressed out by external circumstances. They invariably come down "with the flu." When major losses occur, the loss of a loved one, a divorce, a forced move from home to nursing home, documented evidence exists that these losses at least occasion, if not cause, serious illnesses.[13]

3) Personal Disease. Then comes the disease. Job suffers from a horrible skin disease. He is reduced to sitting on ash or dung and scraping his skin with a potsherd. Job's wife thinks that he has been faithful to God too long, and complains that he should reject God. Job rejects this, remaining faithful: "Shall we accept good from God and not accept evil?"[14] But this initial response is not unwavering.

4) The Lament. The seriousness of his disease now becomes apparent to Job in the poetic sections of the text. People who suffer chronic and serious disease can easily become depressed. The lament focuses on the hopelessness of their life. Job curses the day he was born and yearns for death to release him from his sufferings. Many older people who fall victim to advanced multiple-organ system failure, or advancing senility and the dependency that that causes, have precisely the same feelings.

5) An Appeal to God. Throughout the text, Job continues to appeal to God, rejecting first his friends' arguments that he or his children had sinned so much that God was forced to cause this suffering as retribution. Job later rejects a counselor's fiercer accusations in this regard. Job even fantasizes an afterlife (an uncommon view among the Jews of the period) that allows him to lay his case of innocence before his friends and accusers and before God, Himself. God's justice does prevail.

6) Accusing God. The next step is taken when God does not bail Job out of his dilemma. Then Job's complaints are directed at God. This is the element already cited, of rejecting religion itself.

7) God's Answer/No Answer. Job gets more than he bargained for. God "answers" him out of a whirlwind, but the answer is a reproof. How can Job even think that he can figure out the mystery of the universe? Why we must suffer is one such mystery. God challenges Job: "He who reproves God, let him answer for it" (40:2). Is Job trying to condemn God so he can justify himself (40:8)? At no point does God use the extensive and conventional Wisdom literature explanations so laboriously and confidently argued by Job's friends.

It could be argued that Job's vision of God in a whirlwind is a hallucination. If it is, the parable of Job would not ostensibly change. But the reality of confronting one's own fallible human nature in the presence of the transcendent God would change. Job must "see" God in order for him to understand that he has no real basis for his complaint against God.

8) Surrendering. Job has received his "answer" from God. There is no answer. It is a mystery. One must accept the human condition. One cannot be totally righteous and just. Failure to believe touches all of us in the fearsomeness of God's power in our lives. St. Augustine saw that profundity beyond the sweet and comforting passages of Scripture (see the quote at the beginning of the chapter). Grace is not always a welcome gift.

9) An Experience of God. But *mirabile dictu,* the disaster and the disease have become an experience of God, of God's inscrutable mystery, for Job. Job says: "I had heard of you by hearsay, but now my eyes have seen you. So, I recant and repent in dust and ashes" (42:5–6). God is portrayed as condemning the arguments of those who conversed with Job because they did not "speak the truth of me" (42:7–8).

10) New Blessings. In the Book of Job, Job becomes more prosperous than before, with a new family and flock, blessed by God for going through this trial. It is like a Hollywood ending. In real life, persons might die without vindication or such blessings. But often enough they die reconciled with family and friends, in peace. And that, too, is a blessing.

The essential structure of illness, from a religious perspective, is the almost violent wrenching away from each of us of all the possessions, relationships, and even standards and values that we had assumed were part of our "health." Religious belief teaches us that illness can be a religious experience of the *tremendum;* that real health is found in coming to grips with our own mortality; that the fact that we exist has no ultimate and self-righteous meaning we can construct on our own. Existence is a gift from God and can be taken away: "The Lord gives, and the Lord takes; blessed be the name of the Lord."

A CONTEMPORARY STRUCTURE OF ILLNESS

Leaving the Book of Job for a more contemporary analysis permits us to synthesize the phenomenology of illness in preparation for our discussion of healing in the third chapter.

The state of wounded humanity is a common state. The human experiences of being ill and being healed are ultimately common to all humanity. These experiences themselves help ground our moral commitments, our duties and obligations to one another. The goal of medicine can be formed from what all human beings seek when they seek health.

The essence of the matter is that there are phenomena peculiar to illness that diminish and obstruct patients' capacity to live a specifically human existence to its fullest. These features create a relationship of inherent inequality between two human beings—one a physician (and the rest of the health professionals involved in care), the other a patient. That inequality imposes obligations on the physician. It must be removed as fully as possible before the fullest functioning of the humanity of the person is restored.[15] This is what healing entails.

Those who are ill (that is, those who have experienced some event—a symptom, an injury, a disability—which they regard as "illness") suffer an insult to their whole being. They experience a series of intimate insults to those aspects of their existence that are most integral to being human.

When we become ill, the body is no longer a ready instrument of the will;[16] we lack the knowledge and the skill to make the choices that will restore it; we come necessarily under the power of others, and the integrated image (our embodied selves) that gives meaning to our lives is in consequence shattered. These deficiencies impair the humanity of those who are sick. They become patients, petitioners for help, and the following values incur assaults.

Freedom of Action

One of the essential attributes of being human is the ability to use the body as an instrument of one's own chosen purposes—to attain goals that transcend the needs of the body itself. The body is the human being's instrument for work, play, aesthetic or physical pleasure, and creative activity of every kind. The bodies of plants, by contrast, are rooted and passive. Arguably the bodies of animals are responsive largely to needs that do not transcend the body itself. Locomotion permits a more active pursuit of those bodily needs, and the needs fuel the locomotion. Even if we grant emotional life and emotional satisfaction to higher animals, their bodies do not seem to be instruments of future aspiration or individual creativity. Higher animals pursue happiness, joy, grief, and a loyalty that sometimes appears to human beings to embody altruism (such as dogs or dolphins saving other beings at considerable risk and discomfort to themselves). But to read into this behavior human characteristics may be a form of anthropomorphism.

By contrast, in the human, the body is the agent for highly individualizing and personalizing activities, which serve purposes above and beyond the body itself.

Illness compromises the span of transbodily goals a person may set or attain. The pain, disability, or malaise of illness makes the body the center and end of existence rather than its means. Instead of being commanded, the body itself commands attention. To varying degrees illness moves the patient closer to an animal or even a vegetative existence. Whatever definition we may have given to the "good life," as Job did for his own, must be set aside until the body can be restored as the ready instrument in its pursuit. We must be able to come off the ashheap.

Freedom to Make Personal Choices

The second wound inflicted by illness is the gap in knowledge it opens up, impeding the restoration of health. The sick person lacks knowledge of almost all the essential information and skills needed to heal herself. For example, she does not know what is wrong; she is not sure of how she became ill, or why; she does not know how serious her problem may be, whether she can recover, what treatments are available, whether they are effective, and with what risk, cost, pain, or loss of dignity. She confronts vital choices, yet she lacks the knowledge needed to choose.

The seriously sick person's freedom to make choices and take action in terms of his or her own value system is therefore impaired. The pain, anxiety, and discomfort of illness render the patient susceptible to easy assent to what health professionals may suggest or require. Organic or functional disturbances of the brain add further to this susceptibility. They may even obviate the possibility of free and informed consent or choice, placing the responsibility totally or in part on surrogates. Illness compromises one of the patient's prime and intrinsic characteristics as a human: the characteristic of human agency.

Freedom from the Power of Others

A consistent aim of democratic and humanistic societies is to insure the broadest individual self-determination consistent with the good of all. Each person wishes to be free of the power of others and to enter into personal associations on the basis of freedom and equality. Job is no longer an equal to his friends, as the latter gradually become more strident in offering advice.

In illness this freedom is seriously compromised. Even the most powerful, the most wealthy, and the best-educated become petitioners when they become patients. Marcos could not return to the Philippines, even with all his wealth. Howard Hughes needed Mormon attendants to trim his fingernails during his dying process. Doc Holliday's final words, after all his gunfights, as he lay dying of tuberculosis, expressed the irony of it all: "This is funny." Dependence on professionals, institutions, administrators, technicians—indeed on the whole complex apparatus of hospitals and health care systems—is imposed of necessity upon the sick person.

The power of others to harm and to help inheres in every medical transaction. The patient is at the mercy of the integrity, competence, and motivation of others, most of whom are strangers. In today's complicated, technological health care delivery system, a team is often a necessary and vital aspect of the patient's care. Many team members are never seen, or only fleetingly. Trust must be extended widely—often to unseen persons not bonded to the patient in hands-on care. The dangers of impersonalized use of power are magnified and multiplied as the difficulty in locating responsibility becomes ever more uncertain.[17]

Being ill not only limits the patient's freedom to act and make free choices; it forces her to place trust in others. The resultant vulnerability adds to the patient's plight. Those with the power to heal also have the power to harm or to exploit the patient's vulnerability.

Self-Image

Every illness is an assault on the integrity of the person. The possibilities are sometimes terrifying—survival or death, cure or disability. Pain, discomfort, disfigurement, and limitations loom as possible, probable, or actual. The patient's idea of a satisfying life, one lived according to his own plan, is threatened by the need to adapt to the demand of chronic illness or the threat of recurrent acute episodes.

We are all engaged in a lifelong effort to construct a personal identity—a self-image, like Job's, carefully tailored to balance abilities and limitations. This whole enterprise is eroded by the fact of illness. Illness often demands a drastic reconstruction of image and identity. It challenges self-confidence. The knee-injured linebacker may never be able to play as well again. The overt evidence of vulnerability, often for the first time, is incontrovertible. This is the awesome chasm over which one must leap in faith. A new image, often severely restricted, must be constructed. The patient, after suffering a major heart attack, may have to reduce essential activities. Some patients succeed completely; some succeed only partially; some fail. But all, in some measure or other, must confront the assault on the integrity of the person, concomitantly with the other losses already noted.

More often than not, patients or physicians appreciate the assault as also spiritual. Everything one believed is at risk—especially those prominent belief systems that center on Providence and a personal God. The trials of Job are in one measure or another the trials of every sick person. "Why me O Lord!" "What have I done to deserve this?" "Why now?" "Why not the evil ones of this world?" How often the physician has heard these questions, these laments. They are as unanswerable for modern humankind as they were for Job.

THE WOUNDED HEALER

While we have concentrated in this chapter on the impact of illness and trauma on the patient, there is an analogous impact on the healer as well. The healer hears the questions and they strike into the heart.

First, the healer is bound to the sick person in profound interpersonal and interhuman ways. If this element of the relationship is downplayed, the health professional is victimized, like Job's accuser-friends, by a shortsightedness about things. That same shortsightedness is condemned by Jesus when St. Peter whispers to him that surely he will not suffer the gruesome consequences of his mission, as he has foretold. Jesus snaps: "Get behind me Satan! Your ways are not God's ways." If the physician cannot acknowledge "same-ness" between the patient's sufferings and his or her own, the chance for wisdom, which is understanding and love combined, is severely compromised.

Second, the patient's illness also heals the wounds of the healer. In four separate chants Second Isaiah foresees that the Messiah himself would have to suffer. These are the "Suffering Servant" chants. There are two points to be made here. First, healing comes about in some profound way through the sufferings of others, the sacrifices of others, who themselves must suffer in order to heal. At the very least, health professionals must suffer some ego effacement and some loss of control. The healer, too, must give of himself emotionally, must "suffer with" the sick person. For without a feeling for the predicament of the patient, he cannot truly heal her.

Third, the wounded healer is healed in this process. The physician faces his or her own mortality and comes away from the experience wiser about health, illness, and dying. Almost all older physicians, having faced the death of friends, patients, colleagues, have learned to say good-bye, even as the pain of this lesson increases over the years.

The implications of the healing of the healer will be explored in the seventh chapter, on the community of healing. Suffice it to say at this point that in a pluralistic and relativistic age, a grounding of professional duties and obligations must rest in a reality that transcends cultures and history. The unique impact of being ill on the person, that is to say, the impact on the person's humanity, is by far the most certain source of a humanistic ethics. It is the grounding that gives meaning to the whole of the physician's activities. The need to heal the specific damage done by illness to a patient's humanity imposes moral obligations on physicians.

CONCLUSION: WHY IS IT I WHO MUST SUFFER?

As in the Book of Job, the answer to this timeless question asked by all patients is a mystery. No answer is forthcoming, except that illness is not a punishment from God. It is an opportunity to learn serenity in the face of adversity, to surrender to one's own finitude, to realize that one cannot control one's own body, much less the lives of others. There is peace in this recognition that surpasses understanding. This surrender is not mindless submission. Rather, it is a focusing energy. As Reinhold Niebuhr's Serenity Prayer puts it, it grants "the serenity to accept the things I cannot change, courage to change the things I can, and wisdom to know the difference." Exploring "Why me?" does not lead to a philosophical answer but to a way of life that is dedicated to reality.

NOTES

1. Harold S. Kushner, *When Bad Things Happen to Good People* (New York: Avon, 1983).

2. Hans Jonas, "The Concept of Responsibility: An Inquiry into the Foundations of an Ethics for our Age," in *Knowledge, Value, and Belief*, Vol. 2, *The Foundations for Ethics and Its Relationship to Science*, ed. H. Tristram Englehardt, Jr., and Daniel Callahan (New York: Hastings Center, 1977), pp. 169–198.

3. Soren Kierkegaard, *Either/Or*, ed. and trans. Howard V. Hong and Edna H. Hong (Princeton, N.J.: Princeton University Press, 1987).

4. Edmund D. Pellegrino and David C. Thomasma, *A Philosophical Basis of Medical Practice* (New York: Oxford University Press, 1981).

5. Eric Cassell, "The Function of Medicine," *Hastings Center Report* 7, no. 6 (1977): 16–19.

6. But not Dawson Shultz, who has graciously pointed out this assumption in our own thinking, as it appears in Pellegrino and Thomasma, *A Philosophical Basis*.

7. Galen, *De sanitate tuenda*, I, 5, as cited in Owsei Temkin, "The Scientific Approach to Disease: Specific Saving and Individual Sickness," in *Concepts of Health and Disease: Interdisciplinary Perspectives*, ed. Arthur L. Caplan, H. Tristram Engelhardt, Jr., and James J. McCartney (Reading, Mass.: Addison Wesley, 1981), p. 254.

8. Jurrit Bergsma with David C. Thomasma, *Healthcare: Its Psychosocial Dimensions* (Pittsburgh: Duquesne University Press, 1982).

9. Cassell, "The Function of Medicine."

10. R. A. F. MacKenzie and Roland D. Murphy, "Job," in *The New Jerusalem Biblical Commentary*, ed. Raymond E. Brown, Joseph A. Fitzmyer, and Roland D. Murphy (Englewood Cliffs, N.J.: Prentice-Hall, 1990), pp. 466–488.

11. MacKenzie and Murphy, "Job." The original story of Job was probably contained in the current chapters 1, 2, and 42, the prologue and epilogue. The intervening poetic portion is a later addition to the story.

12. Edmund D. Pellegrino, "The Trials of Job: A Physician's Meditation," *Linacre Quarterly* 56, no. 2 (May 1989): 76–88.

13. See, e.g., Norman Cousins, *The Healing Heart: Antidotes to Panic and Helplessness* (New York: Norton, 1983); and Bernie S. Siegel, *Love, Medicine, and Miracles: Lessons Learned about Self-Healing from a Surgeon's Experience with Exceptional Patients* (New York: Harper and Row, 1988).

14. All quotations are from the *Anchor Bible*, translated with introduction and notes by Marvin Pope (New York: Doubleday, 1982).

15. Pellegrino and Thomasma, *A Philosophical Basis*, pp. 170–191.

16. David C. Thomasma, "*Corpo e persona: Quando scienza e tecnologia travolgono la compassione umana*," *KOS* 5, no. 42 (1989): 6–7, 10–11, 14–15.

17. Edmund D. Pellegrino, "Allied Health Concept—Fact or Fiction?" *Journal of Allied Health* 3, no. 2 (1974): 79–84.

2

Caring and Curing

Although there are many dramatic issues in health care and health care ethics, the most fundamental topic in medical ethics today is the relationship between the person who is ill and those who profess to heal that person—physicians, nurses, the family, the minister, and the social worker. It is the ethical aspects of this relationship that have become so complicated in recent decades. Our discussion in this chapter will deal not so much with the application of specific ethical principles regarding the rights of patients or the duties of health professionals. Rather, we will focus more on the caring than on the curing aspects of the relationship, and on the moral obligations subsumed in the notion of caring. Our next chapter will examine how religion enters the healing relationship through its notion of curing.

We make this distinction because in those two words, "cure" and "care," the recent history of medicine is capsulized. The dominant notion in medicine for most of its history has been caring, even when the physician may have thought that he was curing. Ultimately, curing is a form of caring and one of the most important ways in which physicians do care for their patients. It is only with the introduction of truly scientific means of therapeutics that cure has become possible in any real sense. As a result, the caring aspects of the healing relationship have come to be neglected, and even denigrated.

THE RELATION OF CARING AND CURING

What is the relationship between caring and curing? What are the moral obligations of healers—physicians, nurses, all who come into direct, hands-on contact with sick people?

It is interesting to note at the outset that both words, "curing" and "caring," have the same Latin root, *curo, curare*—"to cure," "to take care of," "to take trouble," "to be solicitous," later becoming "to treat" medically and surgically, "to be devoted to the anxieties and concerns of others," and "to heal" or "restore" to health.[1] The earliest forms of the word meant "anxiety," or "worry." For the greater part of medical history these various senses of curing and caring were essentially one. It is only with the beginnings of truly scientific and therapeutically effective discrete therapies that the possibility of cure without care has existed.

The word "cure" is now often used in a radical sense—to refer to the eradication of the cause of an illness or disease, to the radical interruption and reversal of the natural history of the disorder. In this view a cure restores a patient at least to the state of functioning he or she enjoyed before the onset of the illness, and possibly to even a better state. The possibility of cure in this sense turns on the availability of scientific medicine—radically effective therapeutic modalities that make it possible to "cure" without caring.

Specific, radical, and effective cures, in the technical sense, have become available in the greatest profusion during the lifetimes of physicians who entered the profession following World War II. Before that time, largely through empirical good fortune, some truly effective cures existed (cinchona bark for malaria, foxglove for heart failure, mercury for syphilis), and some were discovered by scientific investigation earlier in this century (insulin, liver extract, sulfonamides). But the golden era of specific therapy has just begun, and its future promises are still to be fully apprehended.[2] We are now in the era of "designer drugs," natural and man-made agents designed to attack the molecular and cellular sources of disease. Surgeons can invade any body cavity to excise, reconstruct, or transplant diseased organs and tissues. Radical cure and restoration—not simply amelioration or disease containment—have become realistic and legitimate goals of medicine.

It is easy, and perhaps some think it desirable, to forget that the greater part of the history of medicine was based on a different meaning of "cure"—that associated with "care" of the ill and sick. To be sure, the extensive pharmacopeias of the Chinese, Indian, and Roman physicians implied curative powers. Some items in them, fortuitously, did cure; most were worthless, or even decidedly dangerous. Cure, if it did occur, resulted largely from the body's self-healing powers and the physician's compassion, caring, encouragement, and emotional support.

The ancient grounding of medicine in care and compassion is seriously challenged by a biomedical model that defines medicine simply as applied biology.[3] In this approach, the primary function of medicine is to cure, and this requires that the physician be primarily a scientist. This model still includes containment of illness by slowing down its progress and by amelioration of its symptoms. But it focuses on *things* to do that are measurably effective for a particular disease, not on the personal involvement of the health care professional in the suffering life of the sick person.

In reaction to this narrow definition, some advocate a broader approach that adds the sociological and psychological to the biological aspects of illness.[4] Others would expand this further to a "holistic" approach, adding religious and spiritual dimensions to the biopsychosocial model. These expanded concepts of medicine imply that all physicians can acquire the requisite understandings and sensitivities the holistic models demand. Such models tend also to absorb all the health professions and a host of related disciplines into medicine, expanding its pretensions beyond all reasonable or responsible hope of fulfillment.

WHAT DOES IT MEAN TO CARE?

Let us now examine what we mean by "caring" and discuss the necessity of a clear concept of its full meaning in understanding the religious foundation of health care and the reformulation of professional ethics. Our comments in this chapter refer to all health professionals, not just to physicians. All are joined in a common task of healing, helping, and caring, and in these endeavors, the same moral obligations bind all similarly.

At root, caring is, as Benner and Wrubel suggest, a "way of being in the world."[5] What they mean by this is that caring is a person's sense of being taken care of therapeutically. By such therapy professionals give patients an identification of what can count as stressful: patients are assured that their experience of stress with disease (being "ill") is all right. But this is not enough. The professional cares therapeutically by identifying coping options that are available. The professional therefore enters into the patient's suffering and helps reconstruct life plans based on values.[6] Thus, caring "is a moral art . . . primary for any health care practice."[7]

At root, however, as Loewy suggests, caring is a biological phenomenon rooted in our emotions and feelings of compassion inseparable from, but not reducible to, the biological substrate of sentient life. While Rousseau talks about even primitive man being endowed with an innate sense of pity, Loewy expands this notion to argue that compassion biologically based is the root of the moral impulse itself.[8]

There are at least four senses in which the word "care" can be understood in the health professions.

Compassion

The first sense is care as compassion—being concerned for another person, feeling, sharing something of his or her experience of illness and pain, being touched by the plight of another person. To care in this sense is to see the person who is ill and at the center of our ministrations as more than the object of our ministrations—as a fellow human whose experiences we cannot penetrate fully but we can be touched by because we share the same humanity. Being touched can only occur if health professionals are open to their own humanity and to its implications in the healing encounter. This can often be the greatest challenge to health professionals.

Activity Replacement

The second sense of caring is to do for another what he or she cannot do for himself or herself. This entails assisting with all the activity of daily living compromised by illness—feeding, bathing, clothing, meeting personal needs—physical, social, and emotional. Physicians do little or none of this kind of care. Nurses do much more, but less than they used to do. A large part of this kind of care is given by nurse's aides in today's team nursing. Yet for most people, loss of the activities of daily living is the biggest rupture of illness in their lives. And replacing those activities, and assisting people to perform them again, is a major element of curing.

Assurance

The third sense of caring is to take care of the problem, to invite the patient to transfer responsibility and anxiety about what is wrong, what can and should be done, to the physician or nurse. This gives the assurance that all appropriate knowledge, skill, and personnel will be directed to the "problem" the patient presents and thereby to altering favorably the natural history of the disease. Assurance includes, but is not limited to, the healing power of the healing professional as a person.

Competence

The fourth sense of caring is to "take care."It is to carry out all the necessary procedures—personal and technical—with conscientious attention to detail and with perfection. This is a corollary of the third sense of care, but it places its emphasis on the craftsmanship of medicine. Together the third and fourth senses are what most health professionals would subsume under the rubric of "competence."

These four senses of "caring" are not really separable in the optimal clinical practice. Nonetheless, in reality, they are often separated, and even placed in opposition to each other. Or caring is reduced to one sense, to the exclusion of the others. For example, the biomedical model of the physician-patient relationship places emphasis on technical competence and conscientiousness, relegating the first two senses—which are more affective than technical—to other health professionals. On the other hand, the expansionist models of medicine—such as the holistic or biopsychosocial—embrace all dimensions of care, blurring the distinctions between them. Partitioning or conflating of the four senses of care leads to either neglect of one aspect or assumption of too much. Both are perilous to the patient.

It is essential that each sense of caring be recognized for its contribution to the healing relationship. Each must be placed in its proper place in an order of priorities determined by the needs of a particular patient. Care is of one piece. The challenge to health professionals is to attend to each sense of care, and so to relate one to the other that they enhance the healing relationship for each patient.

In the ideal healing relationship (patient-physician, patient-nurse) each health professional would attend to each dimension of care in every ministration. When this is not possible—as in contemporary care—these four senses of care must be at least provided by some conscious partitioning of functions among members of the medical or health care team. The moment we make such divisions, we must appreciate that the unity of care is threatened. Special attention must then be given to see that no dimension of care is neglected because none of the health care team members accept the responsibility or see it as proper to their professional tasks or status.[9]

Integral care, that is to say, care that satisfies the four senses we have defined, is a moral obligation of health professionals. It is not an option they can exercise and interpret in terms of some idiosyncratic definition of professional responsibility. The moral obligation arises out of the special human relationship that binds one who is ill to one who offers to help.

THE MOMENT OF CLINICAL TRUTH

All physicians face the conflict between a technically right curing decision and the patient's conception of what is a good decision. In another work, we identified four levels of patient good that enter into clinical decisions.[10] Conflicts arise, for example, when a Jehovah's Witness who can be cured of certain acute situations with a blood transfusion has religious convictions that for him or her precludes that possibility. The right decision technically is not the good decision because it violates the promise that the physician would use his competence for the good of the person who is ill and in a vulnerable state. A person in a vulnerable state is in an unequal relationship in which another has control of his or her life at that moment (the principle of vulnerability will be addressed in chapter 4). Obligations are greatest on the one who has this power in the healing relationship because he or she has voluntarily professed to work for the good of this particular patient.

Cure in the radical sense is not the only aim of medicine. The end of medicine, in the philosophical sense, is a right and good healing decision for a particular human being, a point we made in an earlier book as a centerpiece of the philosophy of medicine.[11] A medically right decision for a patient might be to resuscitate a critically ill patient in the hope that the time gained would eventually lead to cure. The patient may say: "No; I'm not willing to pay that price; I am ready to face death; I am ready to begin the day of my dying." In this case, the right decision and the good decision are in conflict. What we have, then, at the moment of clinical truth is an intersection of value systems, which is the central and focal problem of medical ethics.

This intersection of values must be faced today without the traditional security of a noble, unfailing, universally honored code of ethics.

The recent revisions of the AMA code, the Hippocratic oath, and the other codes derived from it continue to be useful. But they do not face a crucial ethical question of our day—how do we assure that moral choices among and between persons whose values and ethical systems may vary widely can be made in a morally defensible way? How do we preserve our personal moral accountability in a pluralistic society and still assure our patients that we will respect their moral agencies? Without deprecating existing codes, we must recognize that they have lost some of their force because they presuppose a homogeneity of philosophical and even theological values that no longer exists. We have today a plurality of social visions that conflict with one another. With so many differences at so many fundamental levels, is medical ethics doomed to frustrating atomization?

Despite the greater complexity of clinical decisions in a democratic and pluralistic society, the realities of being ill and being healed, or cared for, have not changed fundamentally, and they will not. They are too much ingrained in human existence.[12] To care for the patient in the full and integral sense we have outlined requires a reconstruction of medical ethics, one that attends to the concept of care in its broadest sense and indeed makes caring a moral obligation. This reconstruction must be founded on a moral philosophy that takes into account religious conviction, a unified and integral conception of the community, and an account of what is owed to one another in obligation and love.

REFURBISHING THE IDEAL OF A PROFESSION

The act of profession is the promise health professionals make every time they offer to help a sick person.[13] It declares implicitly to the patient and family that they are competent, that they will use that competence in the interests of the patient, and that they can be trusted not to abuse the privileges that promise entails—to help to manage some of the most significant events in any person's life. It allows them, in the patient's interests, to learn all the weaknesses and foibles, to probe, palpate, prick, and incise the body—a degree of intimacy one does not accord strangers. Sometimes there is more intimacy than there might be in a marriage or other strong bond in society.

No idea has been more debased than the idea of a profession. Today, anyone who undertakes any activity full-time, for pay, or with high skill, anyone who performs some needed service, can call himself or herself a "professional." The list ranges from athletics to astrophysics, from carpentry to car salesmanship, from medicine to mortuary science, from pipe fitting to politics. Whoever is not an amateur, a dilettante, a hobbyist, or an apprentice is accorded the title of "professional."

We have no quarrel with the recognition of excellence in performance, particularly when slovenly craftsmanship is so ubiquitous. Nor do we wish to preserve the term "professional" for some elite purpose. True elitism is not born of titles anyway, but of the voluntary self-imposition of higher than ordinary standards.

Nonetheless, one must not forget that health professionals' act of profession is a declaration of commitment, an act of "consecration," to use Harvey Cushing's word, to a way of life that is not ordinary.[14] In that act health professionals promise that they will not place their own interests first, that they will not exploit the vulnerability of those they serve, that they will honor the trust illness forces on those who are ill.[15] Of course, professionals' real needs can take precedence over the trivial needs of others. Doctors have legitimate self-interests as well.[16] In cases of illness, however, it is not the doctor who has the greatest burden. Because of this imbalance, physicians are required in most instances to place their interests secondary to the patient's. This necessity for a higher standard impelled Plato to use medicine as a paradigm for the ethical use of knowledge.

Later, in the first century A.D., when the word "profession" was first used by Scribonius Largus, it was tied to a special promise of compassion and aid.[17] This has always been the doctor's special promise, the common devotion and the source for his or her ethical obligations. When medicine lacks this ethical dimension, it becomes not just a business, trade, or technique but a betrayal of trust that demeans both the physician and the patient. It is this betrayal that leads to the angry and satirical attacks on physicians so often found in the world's literature. Pomposity, callousness, and cupidity are common human failings. When they are found in physicians, they elicit special rancor because even their severest critics expect better of them.

The most distressing fact is the abuse by some physicians of the trust the nature of their duties demands. Health professionals must merit the trust the act of profession invites. If they do not rise to those obligations, then they can hardly protest when they are satirized, treated as a trade or business, and regulated as such. Moral credibility is theirs to establish and theirs to lose. They cannot blame the Federal Trade Commission, the Congress, the media, or the decline in the general moral standards of society.

The nature of the acts health professionals are expected to perform, together with the trust they demand, forms the basis of professional morality. They bind health professionals even if their philosophical and theological principles differ widely. The professionals are finally responsible for whether their act of profession is a solemn promise, a contract, a commodity transaction, or a business deal. What physicians take the act of profession to be tells more about them than all their rhetoric or codes of ethics.

COPING IN TRUST

Unfortunately, the kind of trust relationship required for so momentous a decision as, let us say, a no-code order (not to resuscitate) is becoming ever more difficult in contemporary medical care. Team care, multiple consultations, rotations of house staff, institutionalization, living wills, fears of litigation, protocols, committees, stress at the moment of decision—all complicate the relationship. In public and teaching hospitals there is often no one with a sufficiently sustained relationship with the patient to serve as a personal physician in the delicate process of making the moral choices true cure and care require. This is a formidable impediment to ethical patient care in the complicated nexus of today's clinical decisions. The reconstruction of medical ethics demands greater attention to the community of healers, as we shall argue in chapter 7.

An ethics of moral decision making must also include respect for the moral agencies and the moral accountability of all health professionals interacting in the clinical decision. The physician may have technical and even legal authority to perform certain acts; the nurse and social worker, others. But no one has moral authority over another, and so all members of the medical and health care teams are morally accountable first to themselves and to their patients. Each promises to help and to act in the patient's best interests. Team decision making is difficult enough. Reaching for "consensus" with others must not be by the abandonment of principles and standards of care.

There will be times when orders cannot be followed because the moral principles of some team members are violated. At other times, if some serious transgression of obligations to patients occurs, "whistle blowing" with all its painful consequences may be necessary. Physicians need far more awareness and sensitivity to the potentialities for moral conflicts with the other health professions and must learn to deal with these conflicts in a way that respects the moral agencies of their colleagues.[18]

It is unlikely that we will ever again enjoy wide agreement on the philosophical or theological sources of our medical morality.[19] It is therefore unlikely that we can achieve general agreement on specific clinical moral decisions. If any common principles are possible, they will probably be deducible only in procedural ethics that respects the obligations of each person to be faithful to his or her own belief system. This is a sad but genuine fact of life in a morally pluralistic society. It must not blind us to one other fact: there are good and bad moral acts. Moral pluralism does not legitimate moral relativism.

How to develop agreement or accord is a most urgent issue in practicing medical ethics in a democratic society. The Hippocratic corpus says very little about the process of making decisions. Rather, it is strongly paternalistic and even warns against sharing information with the patient. The most recent revision of the AMA code is silent on this subject, though it is treated under the heading of consent in the *Opinions of the Judicial Council.*[20] The traditional relationship between doctor and patient has been paternalistic for the most part.[21] When physicians try to become less paternalistic in the process of decision making, some patients object that the doctor "isn't acting like a doctor." Doctors must offer patients autonomy. The patient may decline it. But physicians must not presume that declination and fail to offer it in the first place.

Greater elasticity and openness about who decides is essential. Patients and their families want to know how health professionals will make decisions, who will have the final say, and how we will handle potential conflicts. They will also increasingly want to know the doctor's specific position on such major medical-moral questions as abortion, euthanasia, withholding fluids and nutrition, even access to care.

CONCLUSION

Our moral choices are more difficult, more subtle, and more controversial than those faced when the medical profession acted largely unilaterally. We must not make choices without the heritage of shared values that could unify medical ethics in prior times. Our task is not to abandon hope in medical ethics but to undertake what Camus called "the most difficult task of all, to reconsider everything from the ground up, so as to shape a living society inside a dying society."[22] That task is not the demolition of the edifice of medical morality but its reconstruction along the lines suggested in this chapter: 1) building a specific structure for medical ethics with special emphasis on the ethics of making clinical moral choices; 2) clarifying the "good of the patient" and setting some priority among the several senses, including religious ones, in which that term may be taken; and 3) refurbishing the traditional ideal of a profession as truly a "consecration" of the health professionals' expertise.[23]

The reconstruction we suggest calls upon all in the health professions to attend to the full spectrum of meanings of the word "care." Care is an existential stone in the moral edifice upon which professional obligations are to be re-formed. Caring, instead of being a narrow concept, becomes synonymous with what all healing professionals are about, each in his or her own way. It is also the "common devotion" of all health professionals, the one overriding consideration that should bind in an enterprise that transcends the self-interests of the individual professions.[24]

Normally, a discussion of caring and curing focuses upon specific behaviors that should be extended to individual patients. We have set the discussion of these terms within the moral context of clinical decision making and the reconstitution of the profession. We have done this because one cannot cure and care without attending to the values and to the conception of the good that patients bring to the relationship.

We can now turn to the process of healing itself, in both its historical and its existential contexts.

NOTES

1. "Curo," in *Oxford Latin Dictionary* (Oxford: Clarendon Press, 1983), pp. 473–474.

2. Edmund D. Pellegrino, "The Sociocultural Impact of Twentieth-Century Therapeutics," in *The Therapeutic Revolution: Essays in the Social History of American Medicine,* ed. Morris J. Vogel and Charles E. Rosenberg (Philadelphia: University of Pennsylvania Press, 1979), pp. 245–266.

3. Donald Seldin, "The Medical Model: Biomedical Science as the Basis of Medicine," in *Beyond Tomorrow—Trends and Prospects in Medical Science: A Seventy-Fifth Anniversary Conference (March 8, 1976) [Proceedings]* (New York: Rockefeller University Press, 1977), pp. 31–40.

4. Gerard L. Engel, "The Clinical Application of the Biopsychosocial Model," *American Journal of Psychiatry* 137, no. 5 (1980): 535–544.

5. Patricia Benner and Judith Wrubel, *The Primacy of Caring* (Menlo Park, Calif.: Addison-Wesley, 1989), p. xi.

6. Edmund D. Pellegrino and David C. Thomasma, *For the Patient's Good: The Restoration of Beneficence in Health Care* (New York: Oxford University Press, 1988), pp. 73–91.

7. Pellegrino and Thomasma, *For the Patient's Good.*

8. Erich Loewy, *Suffering and the Beneficent Community* (Albany: State University of New York Press, 1991).

9. David C. Thomasma, "A Code of Ethics for Interdisciplinary Care: A Working Paper," in *Proceedings of the Eighth Annual Conference on Interdisciplinary Health Team Care* (Ohio State University, School of Allied Health Profession and Commission on Interprofessional Education and Practice, Sept. 18–20, 1986), pp. 1–16.

10. Pellegrino and Thomasma, *For the Patient's Good*, pp. 73–91.

11. Edmund D. Pellegrino and David C. Thomasma, *A Philosophical Basis of Medical Practice* (New York: Oxford University Press, 1981), pp. 119–152.

12. The methods of caring for any person who is ill will differ among different societies and tribes, but the root meanings of illness and of caring are universal.

13. Pellegrino and Thomasma, *A Philosophical Basis*, pp. 192–220; Edmund D. Pellegrino, "Toward a Reconstruction of Medical Morality: The Primacy of the Act of Profession and the Fact of Illness," *Journal of Medicine and Philosophy* 4, no. 1 (1979): 32–56.

14. Edmund D. Pellegrino, "The Common Devotion—Cushing's Legacy and Medical Ethics Today," *Journal of Neurosurgery* 59, no. 4 (1983): 567–573.

15. Leon Kass, "Professing Ethically," *Journal of the American Medical Association* 249, no. 10 (1983): 1305–1310; Edmund D. Pellegrino, "Toward a Reconstruction of Medical Morality."

16. Pellegrino and Thomasma, *For the Patient's Good*, pp. 172–189.

17. Georgius Helmreich, ed., *Scribonii Largi Compositiones* (Leipzig: B. G. Teubneri, 1887); Ludwig Edelstein, "Professional Ethics of the Greek Physician," in *Ancient Medicine*, ed. Owsei Temkin and C. Lillian Temkin (Baltimore: Johns Hopkins University Press, 1967), pp. 319–349.

18. The conflict between one's conscience and the need to reach consensus, itself a clinical and team health care problem, is also the principal challenge to holding religious values in a pluralistic society. It is of sufficient importance that it is addressed in later chapters.

19. Alasdair MacIntyre, *After Virtue* (Notre Dame, Ind.: University of Notre Dame Press, 1981).

20. Judicial Council of the American Medical Association, *Current Opinions of the Judicial Council of the American Medical Association* (Chicago: American Medical Association, 1981), p. 25.

21. Pellegrino and Thomasma, *For the Patient's Good*, pp. 11–36.

22. Albert Camus, *Neither Victims nor Executioners*, trans. Dwight MacDonald (Berkeley, Calif.: World without War Council, 1968).

23. Harvey Cushing, *Consecratio Medici and Other Papers* (Boston: Little Brown, 1929), pp. 3–13.

24. Edmund D. Pellegrino, "The Common Devotion."

3

Religion and the Healing Transaction

Does religion enter the healing transaction? Does it influence the ends of medicine and ethical decision making? In what ways?

Whether one takes an existentialist or a principled approach to ethics, religion profoundly influences medicine. Bernard Häring puts it well:

> The whole redemption is a work of healing; therefore the whole of theology, but particularly of moral theology, has an essential therapeutic dimension. Christ the Saviour is also the Healer. He came to heal the individual person in his or her relationships, but he also proclaimed an all-embracing kingdom and therefore a healthful world to live in. Christians are, in Christ, healers. They have a mission to heal themselves, to heal each other and to join hands to create a healthier world.[1]

In this chapter we examine healing and the healing transaction. First we look at the contributions to the healing transaction that religion can bring to medicine, and then discuss the phenomenon of healing. In chapter 7 we will examine the community of healing that is a precondition for the possibility of health care, and the way the community of healing leads to a different perception of the nature of the community from that advanced by libertarian philosophers.

CONTRIBUTIONS TO THE HEALING TRANSACTION

The contributions of religion to the healing transaction are rich and diverse, in anthropology, in the theology of suffering and hope, in the consideration of both body and soul in healing, and in the principle of the intrinsic value of human life.

Anthropology

A religious perspective provides an "anthropology" for medicine,[2] i.e., a theory and perception of the nature of human life. The destiny of human life is paramount in planning for cherished values. This purposefulness grounds the ethical principles of beneficence, justice, and respect for persons.

A religious anthropology grounds beneficence by assisting persons to articulate what they perceive to be the ultimate goal or purpose of their lives as we noted in the first chapter. The experience of one's own life as a gift from God becomes an inherent element of one's attitude toward all interventions in that life. Assessing the physician's recommendations during an illness is part of that attitude. Thus, the patient's view of the good becomes part of the clinical transaction. It does little good to cure a disease if the cure violates the patient's perception of his or her own good.[3]

A religious anthropology also supports justice. It does this by its focus on both the distribution of goods and services for the common good and the care of the vulnerable individual. This is so much a part of the religious viewpoint of healing that Robert Veatch found it challenging to develop a theory of justice toward the vulnerable from a secular point of view.[4] For religious thinkers the common good takes precedence over individual goods, mirroring, as it did for St. Thomas Aquinas, the precedence of the heavenly community over the earthly one. The idea that each person is individually created and cared for by God requires what religious thinkers call "transforming justice." As John C. Bennett says: "By justice I do not mean merely a fair application of existing rules, but a transforming justice that raises the level of dignity and opportunity of all who are neglected and deprived."[5] By this is meant that society itself must be transformed so that the dignity or merit of each individual is secured. This dignity also is to be addressed during illness. Persons working with PWAs (persons with AIDS) constantly point out how difficult it is to sustain commitment and services for these vulnerable individuals. Through their commitment to the person, those who care for AIDS patients must also try to heal society's woeful lack of regard for these suffering individuals.

The third support that a religious anthropology brings to the healing transaction is a grounding of respect for persons. This entails a commitment to protect the values of the individual patient over one's own, even at some risk to "self-interest." On a deeper level, respect for persons is based in a creationist religious vision, that each individual is created by God and is therefore unique and priceless. Sometimes this creation can be interpreted to mean that all human beings are irreducibly and infinitely valuable, since their lives come from God. At other times being created by God is interpreted to mean that all human beings, no matter in what condition, are of equal, intrinsic value. Their lives cannot be judged to be worthless on the basis of external criteria alone, e.g., whether or not they are in a coma, whether they are defective newborns, or whether they are of "value" to society. This is the position represented by the so-called "Seamless Garment" argument, more properly called the "consistent ethic of life," championed by Joseph Cardinal Bernardin.[6] In any event, a religious vision that contains a theology of both creation and redemption will enhance the primary obligation to respect human life, although there may be considerable diversity of opinion about what constitutes proper respect.

A Theology of Suffering and Healing

A religious perspective also proposes that there is a meaning to human existence beyond a person's immediate goals, desires, intentions, and satisfactions. Up through the Middle Ages, and during the Reformation, Christians—both Protestant reformers and Catholics—still embraced a theology of suffering. Sometimes misconstrued or abused, this theology was not always a force for good. But there are important elements that have been lost and must be rediscovered in a proper theology of suffering.

In the older view of suffering, illness was a direct result of sin (especially Original Sin), and healing was a process of reestablishing one's relationship with God. Healing was a matter of the soul. The body, though not neglected, took second place. Part of the reason for this hierarchy is that medicine could not offer for the healing of the body what it can offer today.[7] But another part was, in fact, the perspective of health and illness as a primarily spiritual process. This vision is rare or totally lost today.

This particular conception of healing seems to spring from the thinking of St. Gregory the Great. For Gregory, disease marks "God's correction of human moral, ethical, and spiritual sinfulness."[8] Disease is a sort of chastisement by God to help persons recognize their sinfulness, and help them prepare for a better life. Thus the real disease is located in the soul, and not in the body. This kind of thinking perdured in Jesus' time despite his efforts to decouple sin and illness: "Who sinned, his mother or his father?" he was asked about the blind man. Jesus answered that neither did. Rather the illness is present "to let God's works show forth in him." (Jn 9:2–3).

St. Gregory's view was enshrined in Western civilization. By the time of the Fourth Council of the Lateran, 1215 A.D., the church required physicians to call a priest before attending to the sick. This action was based on the major premise that sickness was often caused by sin.[9] The idea was that once sin was removed, sickness would disappear with the application of medicine.[10] The inheritors of this vision are today's Pentecostal Christians and other religions that eschew medicine almost entirely.

Clearly the ideal was that the sacred and secular, grace and nature, would work harmoniously together. Yet by the sixteenth through eighteenth centuries, Church law required that the patient confess by the third day of treatment by a physician and that a certificate be furnished to that effect. Pius V in 1566 added the following penalty to the Lateran Council rules: "If by the third day, the patient had not confessed and did not furnish a written certificate to that effect, the physician must abandon him; all physicians neglecting this were to be deprived of the doctorate, declared infamous, and fined at the discretion of the Ordinary."[11]

This general attitude led to widespread popular discontent with physicians by the late Middle Ages. Apparently part of the reason for the distrust was that physicians seemed to be greedy. But another part rested on a considerable fear that if they were to focus on healing the body alone, they could do immense damage to the spirit. This would occur if the doctor put the health of the patient's body before the health of the soul.[12] A serious "folly of the sick" was to make use of medicine and not desire the help of God.

Body and Soul in Healing

With the rise of modern scientific medicine, the clash between the religious and secular points of view regarding sickness and health intensified. But the major rupture in Christian anthropology came with the Reformation. The Reform stressed the transcendence of God in human affairs, while the Tridentine reformation of Catholicism stressed the sacramentality or immanence of God. God was so "enfleshed" in the human through Christ that the spiritual and the mundane were wed. Thus, it was expected that sometimes a sacrament of "Extreme Unction" would not only cleanse the soul but also heal the body.[13] The body and the soul, as well as the sacramental realities, oil and grace, were seen as intertwined.

The Reformation view stressed the action of God more than the effectiveness of salvifics. Luther himself suffered many illnesses related to kidney stones, constipation, urinary-tract blockages, and heart disease. While he respected physicians, he retained a sense that illness had a deeper meaning than an attack on the body. He clearly interpreted his own experiences as religious events. Once he became so ill that all vital signs ceased. When he recovered, he penned "A Mighty Fortress," with its stress on the constancy of God and the permanence of God's promise of the Kingdom to human beings: "The Kingdom's Ours Forever."[14]

Calvin proposed a theology in which God has no essential interest in keeping healing works within the Church.[15] His anthropology split the physical from the spiritual, just as Descartes seemed to do. Human beings experience pain and sickness in the mundane world; they experience salvation in a totally other dimension, one, furthermore, that takes primacy over the world of the flesh. Recent studies of the efficacy of prayer during serious illness tend to delimit such clear demarcation between the illness of the body and the healing of the mind. For example, one study found that an IP (intercessory prayer) group in a critical-care unit, though not statistically different from a control group who did not pray together, required less frequent ventilatory assistance, antibiotics, and diuretics than the control group.[16]

The Intrinsic Value of Human Life

Another important principle derived from religion is the doctrine of the intrinsic value of human life. This is a paramount ethical principle, one that both impels human action toward justice and the healing of the disruptions in the community and repels actions such as murder, bombings, and killing the unborn (although this latter is today disputed among religious persons) because these cause disruptions in the community. While there may be secular, philosophical ways of arriving at the same doctrine, these may not be as all-inclusive as a religious argument. The religious argument is based on the belief in a Creator who endows each creature with inalienable rights. It can be a radical power for good or ill in society. [17]

An example of how this principle influences decisions in medical ethics follows. For the most part, positions about withdrawing food and water from patients in serious conditions fall along three lines. First, there are those who argue that such withdrawal may proceed when a person is dying, but cannot when a person is in a stable condition, such as a permanent vegetative state or a permanent coma, or is suffering from Alzheimer's disease in its advanced stages. For this group of thinkers, such conditions do not constitute "dying," and hence, the principles of biomedical ethics regarding the withdrawal or withholding of care cannot apply. [18] To do so would be to "starve and dehydrate" persons to death.

A second set of positions are circumscribed by the principle of autonomy and self-determination. According to these thinkers, a majority of current bioethicists, patients' advance directives (such as a living will) or assignment of a durable power of attorney protect their interests in determining their own treatment when they become incompetent. In this view, it does not matter whether they are dying or not, but what their wishes might be about continued treatment in a perilous condition. Further arguments surround the validity of such advance directives, and whether or not they need to be specific. This was the issue in the Nancy Cruzan case, for example. [19] The problem lay with unspecific preferences about the treatments in question. [20] The heart of the Missouri Supreme Court decision about Cruzan, as well as a New York case about Mary O'Connor, was the specificity of the patient's wishes. [21]

A third point of view can be that the intrinsic dignity of each person requires respect not only for their point of view and their wishes but also for their independence as beings. In this view, it does not matter whether or not a person is dying. What does matter is that no person, no human individual with a spirit, should be subject to any machine or other human intervention without his or her consent. [22] As the Vatican Declaration on Euthanasia puts it:

> One cannot impose on anyone the obligation to have recourse to a technique which is already in use but which carries a risk or is burdensome. Such a refusal is not the equivalent of suicide; on the

contrary, it should be considered as an acceptance of the human condition, or a wish to avoid the application of a medical procedure disproportionate to the results that can be expected, or a desire not to impose excessive expense on the family or the community.[23]

Note how this position entails autonomy of the individual but is more broadly based. It is based in a theory of the healing community, of the rights and responsibilities to others contained in the finite human condition.

A belief in the intrinsic value of human life infuses each of these three positions. As one of us (Thomasma) has argued elsewhere, a fundamental respect for life can assume at least three and probably more contrasting moral positions.[24] The above-named positions also do so. With respect to the healing community, however, they all recognize the basic vulnerability of a sick person. As the Vatican Declaration on Euthanasia underlines: "What a sick person needs, besides medical care, is love, the human and supernatural warmth with which the sick person can and ought to be surrounded by all those close to him or her, parents and children, doctors, and nurses."[25]

We can now turn to the essential features of suffering and healing.

SUFFERING AND HEALING

A religious perspective contributes to an understanding of suffering and healing. Suffering and healing are the privileged places of God's presence in human life. Primarily they are biological phenomena. Suffering prompts human compassion and a primitive sense of pity. And from human compassion in a community arises the way individuals experience God. When persons suffer, they experience:

1. finitude: an intimation of their own mortality
2. vulnerability: an exposure of self to the power of others
3. dissolution: a fracturing of their own personhood
4. disruption: a destruction of normal family and community life

Each of these phenomena can become an opportunity to experience the presence of God's healing power, but each can also lead to despair. The presence and power of God must be offered through the ministry of others. It does not come to persons in isolation as often as to those who have experienced love and sacrifice in families and communities. Healing manifests itself through the community, often in mundane ways. Healing occurs through physical means, from touch to high technology, from combing a patient's hair to heart transplant surgery. On their own, such physical interventions can often cure. But to heal, these interventions must come through other persons. Only persons can effectively heal other persons.

In the debate about active euthanasia, Leon Kass argues that we can be "humane" toward animals precisely because they are animals. We must be "human" toward humans. Thus Kass offers a thoughtful articulation of what is owed a dying patient by the physician. Humanity, he avers, is owed humanity, not just "humaneness," (i.e., being merciful by killing the patient). The very reason we are compelled to put animals out of their misery is that they are *not* human. For animals, there is no theology of suffering that they can create or understand, no "atonement," no reconciliation—in sum, no meaning to suffering. Human beings can develop a theology of suffering for the animals, of course. But animal experience of pain is not the same as human experience. Animals cannot experience the meaninglessness of the pain that is the basis of all suffering, as Viktor Frankl avers. [26]

By contrast, human beings have a claim on our humanity itself. This claim, in turn, rests on the relationship "between the healer and the ill," which is grounded, "even if only tacitly, around the desire of both to promote the wholeness of the one who is ailing." [27] A bond or relationship is created that calls forth a "meaning" for the patient and the healer. Both may create a meaning that relates the experience of pain and its attendant suffering to life plans and ultimate values. A believer may even relate this experience to her own salvation history.

Because healing grows out of the fiduciary relationship of the healers and the one in need, and in and through physical gestures, these gestures acquire an almost sacramental significance. Washing a patient has some features of a sacrament. It is an outward sign of the omnipresence of grace brought to an individual by the community of healers. [28] But so, too, may be cancer chemotherapy, antibiotics, and all other forms of intervention at our disposal. The fact that they are human inventions does not mean they cannot convey God's work. Technology is perfectly capable of being the instrument of an encounter with God.

After all, in eucharistic religious communities, the bread and wine of Communion, which are also works of human hands, are believed to be transformed into God's presence.[29] Technology must be aimed at human goods, of course. But Lazarus is raised from the dead each day in our hospitals. Could this be an interpretation of what Jesus meant about the blind man, that "it was to let God's works show forth in him" (Jn 9: 3)?

Transforming Finitude

In a strict sense, there can be no overcoming of finitude. Each of us must die. Further, each of us carries within a stream of consciousness that is characterized by an awareness of our own finitude, as Heidegger pointed out.[30] As a friend of Jess Lair's exclaimed when Jess had a heart attack and was worried about his forthcoming open-heart surgery: "Ain't nobody, no one of us that's going to get out of this alive, Jess."[31] And as Walt Kelly's Pogo was wont to utter: "We can't be sure we're going to die, but we can be pretty damn sure."[32]

Even though human finitude cannot be surrendered, it can be transformed through creative action by the community. Life, like a sacred torch, is passed on to other generations. Art, music, poetry, sculpture, architecture, and all other forms of human endeavor imitate God's creative and magnificent beauty. Among these forms is the great art of healing, medicine. To be the subject of this art is a transcendent experience.

This point must be taken with caution. The transcendence is not a quality of persons "jumping" out of the limits of the community and the bonds of human finitude. Each sick person is involved in a situation that represents a complex web of interrelationships and habits of mind. Writing of mental health, S. H. Foulkes says something that applies to all illnesses:

> The "situation" is thus a total event, the parts of which add up to something less than the totality; it is constantly in a state of flux; it is a system of relationships displaying a flexible pattern of configurations; and it is organised about some focal point or points which are in reciprocal relationship to each other. . . . The situation is a miniature representation of the world at large which is coterminus and continuous.[33]

Overcoming Vulnerability

Two acts of healing are required to overcome the vulnerability of a patient. The first is that which addresses the need of the patient without regard to the origins of that need. This might be called the nonprejudicial healing of the sick. A good example is our care of alcoholics, AIDS victims, and the many other dispossessed of society. The second vulnerability addressed is the imbalance of power created by that need.[34] The patient has a need that he or she cannot resolve. The healers in the hospital have the power the patient does not possess. In this sense one truly "suffers" (*patior*).[35] To suffer is the root meaning for one who is suppliant, who begs to have a need fulfilled. Since the patient must turn to the community of healers for help, that community has a corresponding duty to respond. This is what is meant by treating "the whole patient." It is also the reason why distinctions cannot be made among patients on the basis of anything but need.[36]

Personhood Reassembled

Caring for a patient's disease does not, in itself, help her resynthesize the dissolution of the person that occurs with illness. In illness, the body phenomenologically stands outside, is alien to the self. It becomes an object, often seen by patients as an object that betrayed them.[37] Even the disease becomes an "it."[38] Because high-quality care is so often identified with high-technology care, there is a great danger that healers will treat the body as an object, too, thus impeding the resolution and restoration of personhood. The aim of all technological interventions, therefore, should not just be their improvement of organ system function. Rather it should include the restoration of personal wholeness through human healing. This is also what is meant by treating the whole person.

Reinserting the Person into the Community

An important element in Jesus' teaching, and indeed in many religions, is that God creates persons to belong to one another in profound and diverse ways and that the bonding of love between persons is equivalent, even identical, to the presence of God. Therefore true healing does not take place until the sick person has been restored to some level of functioning in the community or, if he is dying, until he experiences the compassion and care owed him by his special place as a pilgrim about to complete his journey.

But this feature of restoring individuals in the community may also be derived from secular principles. Clinical experience has shown that some persons do much better than others in coping with serious illness, a point we examined in our previous chapter. This resilience has been studied. For example, burn patients have been encouraged to talk about what helps them cope with tragic and severe trauma. Frequently they cite their religious faith. Encouraging persons to talk about their faith, even if one does not share it, is a crucial way the individual health professional can assist the healing process.[39] It is remarkable how little we speak about what matters the most to patients. Their ultimate values are simply ignored or are considered a matter for the chaplain's service.

Yet talking about the patient's faith, and one's own if it is shared, is a way of respecting the nature of the communities with which we identify in profound and mysterious ways. Even if the faith community is not the matter for discussion, the human community itself ought to be.

Clinicians are surprised that personal faith often leads persons to die more poorly than others who do not have a specific faith. Sometimes this is due to fear of punishment from a *Sturm und Drang* theology in which God is portrayed as angry, graceless, and insensitive from a human point of view. In this instance it may be a challenge to address the deeper aspects of illness and healing we have articulated thus far. The patient may reject all efforts to comfort him.

Historically speaking, we have done poorly with this deeper aspect of healing, even with those who are now cured of their disease. Follow-up care has often been limited to suture removal, prescriptions, taking one's blood pressure, and other activities, often used as a legitimation for *not* engaging the patient's person. It is not sufficient to leave at the doorway of our institutions the commitments to care for persons. Caring begins, not ends, when patients are lifted from their wheelchairs into an automobile. A major task of a hospital is to build communities of care beyond its walls, among the people it serves.

The four elements of healing we just discussed do not exhaust the methods of caring for persons that can function as the "outward signs" of grace. One might consider that healing is a "sacrament," analogous to and expanded upon a more vigorously exercised sacrament of the Anointing of the Sick. In this reconstitution, note that the ministers of this analogous sacrament are all those persons who "lay hands" on the patient, whether through the medium of medical interventions, technology, or less intensive activities. Thus, a minister of this "sacrament of healing" might be the woman who washes the floor of the room and talks to the patient while doing so, the nurse's aid who combs the patient's hair, the sister-chaplain, the non-Catholic billing clerk, and so on. If anything, healing is an ecumenical sacrament. [40]

In this new vision, the ministers may be those ordained by their skill, knowledge, and commitments to care for the sick. They are sealed by grace through their calling to heal rather than just to cure. Because all persons have been redeemed by God through the cross, all persons may have access to this healing gift, even if they cannot all gain access to specifically expensive forms of health care.

But how does the clinical event become such an analogous sacrament? A sacrament is an outward sign that gives grace. Recall the discussion of Christ's proclamation of the reign of God through his healing ministry. The public sign of healing is also effective. It brings about the rule of God just as it announces it. Thus, the clinical event first and foremost becomes a saving event if the intention of the healer is to imitate what Christ did as a sign of sacrificial love, a love that joins the participants together with Christ. As Lambourne states: "The making of the clinical event a salvation event is to diagnose it as a predicament of wrong relations between man and man, and man and God."[41]

Second, and most important, the sacramental healer must believe in the reconciliation made possible by God's grace. If healing is brought about by those who do not believe or do not share in the explicit faith commitments of religious institutions, the intention itself could be seen as lodged in the commitments of the community of healers, the spiritual dedication of the institution's members as a whole, and, of course, in the beliefs of the patient who seeks to be healed. Reconciliation may still take place, but it is not a specific feature of healing, as might appear in a quasi-sacramental healing encounter.

CONCLUSION

Religion and religious commitment are essential components of healing for many people. For unbelievers different components may come into play in the healing process. Religious commitments contribute to healing by providing an anthropology, a theology of suffering and of healing, asserting the intrinsic value of human life as the basis for the role of the community in healing.

Even for nonbelievers, illness, the confrontation with finitude and suffering, must be faced on something other than the biological level. Illness is intensely personal and yet effectively communal. In this sense, therefore, all illness, healing, and coping transcend technology and call forth effort to assist in coping, in adjusting one's life plan, self-image, and spiritual existence.

NOTES

1. Bernard Häring, *Free and Faithful in Christ*, vol. 3 (New York: Crossroad, 1981), p. 1.

2. Note that we use the term "anthropology" in a philosophical sense here, as a theory of the nature of human being and human life.

3. Edmund D. Pellegrino and David C. Thomasma, *For the Patient's Good: The Restoration of Beneficence in Health Care* (New York: Oxford University Press, 1988), pp. 73–126.

4. Robert Veatch, *The Foundations of Justice* (New York: Oxford University Press, 1987).

5. John C. Bennett, "Ethical Aspects of Aging: Justice, Freedom, and Responsibility," in *Ethics and Aging*, ed. James E. Thornton and Earl R. Winkler (Vancouver: University of British Columbia Press, 1988), p. 41.

6. Joseph Cardinal Bernardin, *The Consistent Ethic of Life* (St. Louis: Catholic Health Association, 1988).

7. James E. Rush, *Toward a General Theory of Healing* (Washington, D.C.: University Press of America, 1981), pp. 80–92.

8. Rush, *General Theory of Healing*, p. 85.

9. Rush, *General Theory of Healing*, p. 89.

10. Henry C. Lea, *A History of Auricular Confession and Indulgence* (Philadelphia: Lea Brothers, 1896), p. 262.

11. Lea, *Auricular Confession*, p. 263.

12. Darrel Amundsen, "The Medieval Catholic Tradition," in *Caring and Curing: Health and Medicine in the Western Religious Traditions*, ed. Ronald L. Numbers and Darrel W. Amundsen (New York: Macmillan, 1986), p. 91.

13. Marvin R. O'Connell, "The Roman Catholic Tradition since 1545," in *Caring and Curing*, ed. Numbers and Amundsen, pp. 108–145.

14. Carter Lindberg, "The Lutheran Tradition," in *Caring and Curing*, ed. Numbers and Amundsen, pp. 173–203.

15. Rush, *General Theory of Healing*, p. 91.

16. Randolph C. Byrd, "Positive Therapeutic Effects of Intercessory Prayer in a Coronary Care Unit Population," *Southern Medical Journal* 81, no. 7 (1988): 826–829.

17. David C. Thomasma, *Human Life in the Balance* (Louisville: Westminster Press, 1990).

18. Eugene Diamond, *This Currette for Hire* (Chicago: ACTA Foundation, 1977).

19. Society for the Right to Die, *Right-to-Die Backgrounder* (New York: Society for the Right to Die, 1989).

20. Society for the Right to Die, *Backgrounder*, p. 2.

21. Society for the Right to Die, *Backgrounder*, p. 15.

22. This is the central thesis of Thomasma, *Human Life in the Balance.*

23. Sacred Congregation for the Doctrine of the Faith, *Declaration on Euthanasia* (Vatican City: Polyglot Press, May 5, 1980) as reproduced in The President's Commission for the Study of Ethical Problems in Medicine and Biomedical and Behavioral Research, *Deciding to Forego Life-Sustaining Treatment* (Washington, D.C.: United States Government Printing Office, 1983), p. 306.

24. Thomasma, *Human Life in the Balance.*

25. Sacred Congregation for the Doctrine of the Faith, "Declaration on Euthanasia," *Vatican Council II* 2 (1982): 510–16 at 516, as reprinted in Kevin O'Rourke, O.P., and Philip Boyle, O.P., *Medical Ethics: Sources of Catholic Teaching* (St. Louis: Catholic Health Association, 1989), pp. 109–110 at 110.

26. Viktor Frankl, *Man's Search for Meaning* (New York: Simon & Schuster, 1984).

27. Leon Kass, "Arguments against Active Euthanasia by Doctors Found at Medicine's Core," *Kennedy Institute of Ethics Newsletter* 3, no. 1 (1989): 1–3, 6. This article is a shorter version of "Neither for Love nor Money: Why Doctors Must Not Kill," *Public Interest* 94 (Winter 1989): 25–46.

28. We will examine the community of healers in more detail later.

29. David C. Thomasma, *An Apology for the Value of Human Life* (St. Louis: Catholic Health Association, 1983), pp. 95ff.

30. Martin Heidegger, *Being and Time*, trans. John Macquarrie and Edward Robinson (Oxford: Blackwell, 1973).

31. Jess Lair, *I Ain't Much Baby, but I'm All I've Got* (New York: Fawcett Books, 1985).

32. Walt Kelley, *I Go Pogo* (Hastings-on-Hudson, New York: Ultramarine, 1977).

33. Siegmund H. Foulkes and E. James Anthony, *Group Psychotherapy* (New York/London: Penguin Books, 1957), p. 30.

34. Edmund D. Pellegrino and David C. Thomasma, *A Philosophical Basis of Medical Practice* (New York: Oxford University Press, 1981), pp. 155–169.

35. "Patior, pati, passus sum," in *Oxford Latin Dictionary* (Oxford: Clarendon Press, 1983), pp. 1309–1310.

36. Pellegrino and Thomasma, *A Philosophical Basis*, pp. 170–191.

37. Jurrit Bergsma with David C. Thomasma, *Healthcare: Its Psychosocial Dimensions* (Pittsburgh: Duquesne University Press, 1983).

38. Eric Cassell, "Disease as an 'It,'" *Social Science and Medicine* 10 (1976): 143–146.

39. Kimberly A. Sherrill and David B. Larson, "Adult Burn Patients: The Role of Religion in Recovery," *Southern Medical Journal* 81, no. 7 (1988): 821–825.

40. Robert A. Lambourne, *Community, Church, and Healing* (London: Darton, Longman & Todd, 1963), pp. 87–90. Lambourne argues that the sacrament of mercy and healing should not be confined to the believing society of the Church. The ubiquity of acts of mercy among all humans means that the notion of the Church (as we have argued) and the community should be expanded to include "the fullness of Christ." Lambourne, p. 88, says: "These acts [of mercy] can, by the word of God, be made salvation events, so that the pagan social worker or surgeon may provide the form, as the bread or wine, and the Christian witness the word at quite another time and place. Together they make one sacrament which offers salvation to both Christian and non-Christian about the clinical event." Lambourne acknowledges that this "universalistic aspect of the cup of cold water" would change and expand the concept of all sacraments, just as in Mark 10, when John asks about the unauthorized man healing in Jesus' power.

41. Lambourne, *Community, Church, and Healing*, p. 86.

4

The Principle of Vulnerability

In 1988, Pope John Paul II came to the United States for a second time. During that trip he visited an AIDS hospice. His talk on that occasion challenged Catholic health care with a special mission to the outcasts of our society, and especially to those persons who suffer from AIDS. This challenge is a good example of the "healing community" principle to be enunciated in chapter 7. According to this principle, there is a "special mission" in religious health care to the most vulnerable in society. We saw in the previous chapters how such a special mission might be based upon a religious experience about illness and the intimation of our own mortality, to which we can only surrender. It is not so much acceptance as an awareness of finitude. And this awareness concerns not only our lives but also our values and standards, our possessions and relationships. What we, patients and health professionals alike, discover is that we are all vulnerable.

In this chapter we will focus on the thread of vulnerability that has run throughout our reflections thus far. Vulnerability grounds the awareness of common bonds and the duties of health professionals to heal. It moves us beyond curing to caring and assists religiously inspired health professionals to protect their principles in a morally pluralistic society.

VULNERABILITY AS A PRINCIPLE: GENERAL ETHICS

In a previous work we derived a concept of vulnerability from the nature of medicine as a special kind of human activity.[1] We held that to attain the goal of the medical encounter—a right and good healing action for a particular patient—several axioms were necessary, the violation of any one of which imperils the goal. Observing the vulnerability principle was one of these necessary axioms.

It could be derived from other sources as well. A good argument for treating the vulnerability of individuals might be constructed using the principle of respect for persons. Those who become vulnerable for one reason or another would command special respect. We prefer to ground it, as Loewy does, in the capacity to suffer. He argues that the common capacity to suffer confers prima facie rights not to be caused suffering, that the community is primarily concerned with beneficence in which autonomy emerges, and that thus the community has an obligation not only to refrain from causing suffering but also to ameliorate suffering and prevent its occurrence among its members. The social contract in Loewy's thought arises from this capacity to suffer, in that solidarity in community arises from individuals' perceptions that the community contracts with them to address their suffering and tries to prevent it.[2]

The principle of vulnerability can be stated this way: in human relations generally, if there are inequities of power, knowledge, or material means, the obligation is upon the stronger to respect and protect the vulnerability of the other and not exploit the less advantaged party. This is a principle of general ethics, applicable to all sorts of human relationships. It generates an obligation of altruism, i.e., taking others into account in our use of power, knowledge, or other possessions. This taking of vulnerability into account is a bilateral or a multilateral affair.

Goodin, in his *Protecting the Vulnerable*, analyzes important cases regarding the vulnerable in contracts, business relations, professional ethics, family relations, among friends, and in relationship benefactors.[3] He builds an inexorable case in social justice that society bears specific responsibilities toward those who, in any particular relationship, are more vulnerable to exploitation or harm. The heart of his argument is that we usually assume that the basis for special responsibilities to protect the vulnerable from harm come from self-assumed duties and obligations, often through contracts, implied or explicit. A good example of the former might be the obligation of families to provide for their children first, over caring for others in society,[4] or the obligation of a health professional for his or her own patient over other needy persons in society, as Veatch argues.[5]

This assumption is probably wrong, according to Goodin. Rather than being grounded in contracts by which we voluntarily commit ourselves to a limited range of persons (as the libertarians would have it), the obligation is grounded in the vulnerability of the persons themselves: "Examining several cases closely, however, suggests it is the *vulnerability* of the beneficiary rather than any voluntary commitment per se on the part of the benefactor which generates these special responsibilities."[6] The beauty of this argument rests on real cases that have been adjudicated in American courts. A secular principle grounded on suffering can supply such obligations. Religious views may or may not reinforce this grounding; some religions may—and others may not—see in vulnerability the road to redemption.

The conclusion reached by Goodin is based upon how we actually behave, how our deepest values, expressed in our social thought and jurisprudential theory, are brought to bear on individual persons in conflict in our society.

Vulnerability and Justice

A secular principle of justice cannot easily supply any special moral obligations to care for certain segments of the population, even if they are so obviously suffering. The vulnerability principle, while developed in various ways in philosophical and political literature, is also a religious principle of justice. As St. Augustine articulated it long ago, "to each according to his need" is the basis of a committed community.[7]

Furthermore, if vulnerability is, indeed, the basis of responsibilities, then many more people are vulnerable with respect to us. Since special responsibilities toward certain groups within society are one our firmest moral intuitions, then this moral intuition must also embrace all those others who are vulnerable but fall outside our "normal" understanding of those to whom we are specially responsible.

The problem with the above argument, that vulnerability is the basis of responsibilities, is that the social thought and jurisprudential theory can be counterargued by those who Hume said had "limited benevolence" in society.[8] We are all too familiar with the "me, too" generation, the social narcissism that infects our society, and the strident calls for autonomy and individualism.[9] For persons with this view, there is no duty that is not explicitly and freely accepted by individuals. That people are vulnerable or poor or downtrodden or disvalued is unfortunate but not unjust. Persons who have not directly caused such problems are not responsible for their solution, unless they voluntarily assume those responsibilities. Indeed, Rawls's arguments for social duties in justice are based on a theory of self-interest. Behind a veil of ignorance about our own eventual social standing, we would be impelled to altruism to protect our own needs and interests.

That is why David Ozar argues that it is insufficient, in terms of social justice, to concentrate merely on the rules governing good contracts to fulfill our obligations. At the base of all contracts and covenants between persons is a duty to right any imbalance within those contracts.[10]

But where does this claim come from? Can it be sustained philosophically? The only way it may is by social agreement about the nature of human society itself. Originally, Western society was infused by a religious vision of the interrelationship of individuals. But as this religious foundation eroded, agreement about what constitutes a good society was gradually lost. The principle of vulnerability found itself embodied in philosophical theories of social justice. Rawls, for example, argues that we must protect peoples' "needs," "primary goods," or "vital interests."[11] This duty applies even despite differing social judgments regarding those needs and vital interests.

Vulnerability and the Religious Perspective

We already noted that many thinkers place the philosophical basis for protecting the vulnerable in a social contract, in and through which reasonable people try to protect their own self-interests. "Enlightened self-interest" was one of the catchwords of the sixties, whereby businesspeople and politicians "bought into" the civil-rights movement because boycotts and the threat of boycotts hit them in the pocketbook. This pragmatic corrective to the alternative, social chaos, fits entirely into John Adams's theory of the ideal republic being a "mixed polity." By "mixed polity," as Andrew Reck argues, Adams meant a polity in which the natural law balanced "the classes of mankind in the structure of government in order to assure political stability and to escape the cyclical overthrow of governments destroyed by the vices of corruption that otherwise go unchecked."[12] Thus, from the point of view of natural reason, caring for the most vulnerable in society can be grounded in a theory of checks and balances that avoid, for example, the unraveling of civilization such as in Liberia in 1990 or in other societies in which governments wallow in corruption. Another argument for the obligation to care for the most vulnerable can be derived most clearly from a religious perspective. In this view, all individuals are created by God. As one consequence, their fundamental goods, including, most of all, life itself, are to be protected. Each person has inherent value, despite what external valuations society might place on him or her. This is the origin of the "preferential option for the poor" that obligates institutions and individuals to reach out first to the most needy before caring for other persons.[13] The vulnerability of those who are social outcasts as well as ill—persons with AIDS, the poor, the weak and debilitated elderly—is a call to charity and solicitude. Vulnerable persons become the "deeded suffering." They can expect from those with a religious commitment help in relieving their sufferings of indignity and neglect. In a modern, secular, or libertarian society, their vulnerability is considered to be unfortunate, but it generates no obligations on those who are better off.

The Kingdom preached by Jesus is a spiritual entity within each human being and a visible entity manifested in the lives and conduct of believers.[14] The Resurrection is partially fulfilled in the present. We are already living the resurrected life. Our recognition and affirmation of the Resurrection and the love it entails should be manifest in our health care institutions to all people in need.

The Catholic Church in the United States has advanced the premise of the intrinsic value of every human being through its various human-life campaigns. This is especially true of its "consistent ethic of life," adopted unanimously by all the Catholic bishops.[15] Popularly called the "Seamless Garment" argument, the consistent ethic of life proposes that a belief in the creative and redemptive acts of God requires an inherent respect for all forms of human life, from fetuses to enemies, to the poor, and so on. Some difficulties exist with this premise. Should a consistent ethic of life target only the vulnerability of human life, or should it include animal life as well, or environmental ethics? Further, are all forms of human life to be considered of equal merit from the point of view of W. D. Ross's prima facie obligations?[16]

That being noted, a narrower human-life ethic has sometimes been a linchpin for too negative a definition of Catholic health care. All too often, the Christian identity of a facility has been based on what it does *not* do (abortions, sterilizations) than what it *does* do. The broader conception of devotion to each human person regardless of status or friendship with the caregivers is a more profoundly Christian basis for the Christian health care mission. A leading influence in this direction is the Christian personalism of Karol Wojtyla himself.[17]

A major way to describe a vision in contrast to secular points of view about caring for the vulnerable is that of the "committed institution." We coin this phrase to describe the incredible ability of the Christian tradition to institutionalize its goals, commitments, visions, and aspirations. The Catholic Church, for example, is regarded even by its critics as especially adept at organization. Institutions crystallize momentary callings in a more permanent form so that they will endure after the deaths of the visionaries who inaugurated the movement.

This tendency to institutionalize a vision can be both a strength and a weakness, a joy and a curse. One can find comfort in such structures, or agony when they need reform. One method of building on the strength of this tradition, however, is to make health care institutions more explicit about what they stand for in the community, what conduct can be expected by patients from reading the institution's mission-and-philosophy statement. Thomasma has argued elsewhere that hospital ethics committees can help fulfill this function by providing a forum for individual practitioners in the institution to form its conscience and help proclaim this to the community.[18] Pellegrino has argued for the collective moral responsibility of the hospital board of trustees and staff—a responsibility built upon a promise of service to a community.[19]

VULNERABILITY AS A PRINCIPLE: HEALTH CARE ETHICS

Vulnerability is a common feature of many human relationships, but it has a special urgency in the healing relationship. Here both the healer and the person being healed are vulnerable, each in different ways, defined by the power each may exert over the other.[20]

We have detailed in earlier works and in the present effort the vulnerability of sick persons. A central phenomenon of illness is the vulnerability of the sick person and the consequent inequality it introduces into the medical relationship. Even the most self-sufficient person becomes anxious, fearful, and dependent when illness occurs. Patients lose freedom to pursue life goals, to make their own decisions, and to heal themselves without access to specialized knowledge and skill. Pursuit of relief, a cure, and a return to health becomes the central preoccupation. In this state the sick person is forced to consult another person who holds the needed knowledge and skill and who therefore has power over the ill person. The heart of this power lies in the fact that the patient is unable to judge the competence of the physician, the doctor's advice or operative skills. The ill person must in this state seek help from the physician and trust him or her at some point.

These facts impose a condition of inequality on the medical relationship paralleled by few other situations in democratic societies. Taken together, they add up to a state of unusual vulnerability and susceptibility. This inescapable vulnerability imposes de facto moral obligations on the physician. In a relationship of such inequality the weight of obligations is on the one with the power. This is very different from the ethos of business, where vulnerability is an opportunity to exploit one's adversary. On the contrary, the physician has the obligation to protect the patient's vulnerability against exploitation. She is obliged to be faithful to the trust that is ineradicable in medical relationships. When she offers to help, the physician elicits trust that she will act for the good of the patient, not self-interest, the good of society, science, the family, or any other entity. The ethos of the profession must somehow synthesize public and private good, both of which are needed for social good but not for the private, egotistical good of the individual.

Dehumanization

Dehumanization is created in part by the impersonality of modern society. In medicine it is also created by the increasing reliance upon technological interventions to cure persons, rather than personal reaching out by the healer toward the person to be healed. Both patient and physician suffer in this regard. The exquisite irony of dehumanization is evident when one enters a patient's room and finds nurses and doctors fussing more over the machinery than over the patient hooked to the machine. This is necessary, of course, if technical care is to be administered properly. But health care professionals can become slaves to the technology instead of being servants of the patient.

Of greater concern is that the technology is applied either sloppily or without attention to other levels of values that the patient and family may bring to the clinical encounter. If it is sloppily applied, ethical issues arise immediately. If no attention to other values is paid, individuals feel betrayed by the promise to heal.

Specialization

The increasing specialization of health care personnel creates opportunities for clashes among professionals, genuine disputes about proper patient care decisions. But more important, technical care creates a division of labor that can degenerate into partitioning the patient into organ systems, functions, and body parts. Individual attention to persons in need becomes more and more difficult. With the decline of the general physician, it is often difficult to know who is in charge, who will "bring it all together," when the patient is in the hospital setting.

Andre Hellegers, the founder of the Kennedy Institute of Ethics, warned prophetically years ago:

> As the caring branches of medicine were gradually pushed aside by the curing ones, there seemed to be less use for the Christian virtues. I think that shortly the need for those old Christian virtues will return and once again be at a premium. Our patients will need a helping hand and not a helping knife. This is no time to dismantle the low-technology care model of medicine. . . . We must either recapture the Christian virtues of care or we shall be screaming to be induced into death to reach the "discomfort-free society."[21]

Institutionalization

The growth of specialization and technology has meant that more and more care must be delivered in and through institutions. Institutions characteristically have laws, structures, and procedures. Often these infantilize persons, especially the elderly and disabled. As a result, many of the patients' most important values are submerged or violated. For example, persons in institutions are often automatically regarded as candidates for CPR unless they explicitly request a Do Not Resuscitate status. This decision by default means that patients will be resuscitated unless there is an order to the contrary. Without question this may help save some lives, particularly in the emergency room. But is also creates the modern counterpart of ancient tragedies, unduly prolonging the act of dying.

But institutionalization also affects the hospital staff. The emphasis on technology and institutionalization often makes it possible for individuals to defect from their obligations as moral agents in favor of the rules of the institution. When this is combined with the dominion of autonomy as a legal and moral primary principle, physician and nurse may feel absolved from responsibility for the welfare of the patient.

Dying by Whim of Others

Keeping a person alive at all costs is a form of biological idolatry. This idolatry denies the finitude of human existence and feeds the illusion of immortality that medical prowess seems to dangle before us. It also encourages the erroneous assumption that "good" care is synonymous with unrelenting high-technology medicine. Some even see it as a form of hostility on the part of the caregiver.[22] Healing, to be fully effective, must be a ministry of persons, not of technology. This means that patients and doctors must not be overshadowed by technology. Technology must always be directed to the good for human beings. Dying, like living, is a personal matter, not a problem to be "solved" by formula, mechanical means, or even well-intentioned efforts to coerce the patient's choices.

Social Parsimony

To these sources of vulnerability we must add the context of a growing attitude of social parsimony for health care and other fundamental human needs. So many nations exhaust their resources in expenditures for armaments, in mismanagement or bureaucratic corruption, or in pursuit of mindless amusements that the care of the sick is compromised, ignored, or even denigrated. The principle of vulnerability has no chance of survival in a mean-spirited, belligerent, ethnocentric climate.

All of this goes to the heart of the theological question: what sort of society ought we to be? This question is not only conceptual. It requires a social commitment to some notion of a good society and determination to shape public policy toward this end. Conceptual analysis helps to shape our attitudes toward social policy. But the analysis is only propaedeutic to social change. And social change occurs only in the context of a perspective beyond the one currently in vogue, usually one that touches the most basic elements of our shared humanity.

A life-affirming society ought to base its public policy in health care on personalist principles. A good public policy in health care is one that empowers physicians, other health workers, and patients to enter a healing relationship that meets the needs of the individual within the community of healing—one that in essence takes seriously the obligations that grow out of the vulnerability of the sick.

The precise configuration of a public policy that might foster a life-affirming society is a complicated subject outside the purview of the present work. Each of us has made suggestions about the criteria that might be morally defensible in constructing public policies of resource allocation, or rationing, should that become a practical necessity.[23] Suffice it to say that we would oppose policies that discriminate on the basis of age,[24] social status, social worth, ability to pay,[25] or laissez-faire market economics.

A society reveals its most fundamental values in the way it distributes its resources among the most vulnerable of its members. Especially in a society that claims to take much of its ethos from Christianity, nothing less will do than to distribute those resources in accordance with the principle of charity, in the spirit, if not the letter, of the Sermon on the Mount. Other religious worldviews have ordering principles that govern their attitudes toward their most vulnerable members. While there will be differences of detail among religious perspectives, all, if faithfully lived, would reject the market mentality and commercial spirit that have gained so much support in the socially parsimonious climate of health care today.

THE MISSING PERSPECTIVE

Coherent theorizing about health care lacks determination and resolution unless it is informed by reality. The doctor and the patient, the hospital and the nursing home, Medicare and Medicaid—all exist within the context of political pressures to cut back commitments to care, and of a pragmatic social environment obsessed with power and the powerful. Out of this environment comes the mixed message: "Yes, persons are important. Yes, there is a value to human life. But no, this particular person is 'too far gone' to worry about. No, this old person should no longer receive care."

One way vulnerable persons have been protected in the past has been through the commitments of traditional medical ethics. The enormous burst of energy that characterizes biomedical ethics in the last two decades has exposed a vast array of new, complex, and largely unresolved problems.[26] The predominant mode of ethical discourse has been philosophical and analytical, procedural rather than normative.[27]

Valuable as this approach has been in raising sensitivities among health care professionals and changing professional practices, it suffers from the lack of a coherent moral philosophy and theology of medicine upon which to ground its principles, duties, rules, and virtues. It does achieve the limited aim of agreement on certain points, but it submerges, without eradicating, the deeper moral sources—religious or secular—from which the entire rational superstructure of medical ethics has originated.

The deficiencies we perceive in contemporary biomedical ethics are the deficiencies of a dialectical rhetoric without a moral philosophy or some set of ordering principles bequeathed us in religious belief to resolve conflicts or elucidate principles, duties, and obligations. The result is an increasingly cacophonous debate, increasingly divisive and alarmingly atomistic.

Public policy today too often stresses individual rights to the detriment of the community's values. More important, it stresses the rights of power over the protections we ought to place on the increasing vulnerability of the ill, the tired, the depressed, the aged, the poor, and the outcast. We support wholeheartedly the protection of individual rights and the dignity of human persons that gives rise to the principle of autonomy. We hold, however, that a religious perspective requires that more is owed to the most vulnerable among us. Invoking autonomy is not an excuse for shirking beneficence. Properly ordered societies in the developed world, at least, can protect individual freedom as well as be solicitous of the special needs of each when the vulnerability inherent in illness manifests itself.

CONCLUSION

How we interpret the same principles—autonomy, justice, and beneficence, for example—depends very much on what theory of ethics we espouse and, even more significant, on where we seek the ultimate sources of morality. These sources may be biological determinism, social custom, historical precedents, philosophical inquiry, scriptural texts, attempts to resolve conflicts in texts, revelation, Church teachings, or traditions. How we justify our conduct toward the needy will depend heavily on which sources we use. This, the deepest and most firmly embedded level of moral discourse, is in the long term the most influential, the most sharply divisive, yet the most often neglected level of debate about public policy.

Society built on Christian ethics should protect the most vulnerable from harm. Toward them more should be given than toward those with power. This is what we think Jesus meant when he said: "The last shall be first, and the first, last."

NOTES

1. Edmund D. Pellegrino and David C. Thomasma, *A Philosophical Basis of Medical Practice* (New York: Oxford University Press, 1981), pp. 155–169.

2. Erich Loewy, *Suffering and the Beneficent Community* (Albany: State University of New York Press, 1991).

3. Robert E. Goodin, *Protecting the Vulnerable* (Chicago: University of Chicago Press, 1985).

4. Goodin, *Protecting the Vulnerable*, pp. 4–5. As he points out, sociobiologists claim that our genetic makeup itself may dictate that we confine "reciprocal altruism" rarely narrowly to the family. See R. L. Trivers, "The Evolution of Reciprocal Altruism," *Quarterly Review of Biology* 46 (1971): 35–57; Matthew Ridley and Richard Dawkins, "The Natural Selection of Altruism," in *Altruism and Helping Behavior,* ed. J. Philippe Rushton and Richard M. Sorrentino (Hillsdale, N.J.: Lawrence Erlbaum Associates, 1981), pp. 19–39; Peter Singer, *The Expanding Circle* (Oxford: Clarendon Press, 1981).

5. Robert M. Veatch, *The Foundations of Justice* (New York: Oxford University Press, 1986); Robert M. Veatch, *A Theory of Medical Ethics* (New York: Basic Books, 1981).

6. Goodin, *Protecting the Vulnerable*, pp. xi, 42–108.

7. St. Augustine of Hippo, *The Rule of St. Augustine* (London: Darton, Longman & Todd, 1985).

8. David Hume, *An Enquiry Concerning the Principles of Morals* (Indianapolis: Hackett, 1983).

9. H. Tristram Engelhardt, Jr., *The Foundations of Bioethics* (New York: Oxford University Press, 1986).

10. David Ozar, "The Social Obligations of Health Care Practitioners," in *Medical Ethics: A Guide for Health Professionals,* ed. John Monagle and David C. Thomasma (Frederick, Md.: Aspen, 1988), pp. 271–280.

11. John Rawls, *A Theory of Justice* (Cambridge: Harvard University Press, 1971).

12. Andrew J. Reck, "Natural Law and the Constitution," *Review of Metaphysics* 42, no. 3 (1989): 503.

13. Laurence O'Connell, "The Preferential Option for the Poor," in *Medical Ethics,* ed. Monagle and Thomasma, pp. 312–317.

14. John Sanford, "The Puzzle of the Kingdom of God," in *Afterlife: The Other Side of Dying*, ed. Morton Kelsey (New York: Crossroad, 1985), pp. 274–289.

15. Joseph Cardinal Bernardin, et al., *The Consistent Ethic of Life* (Kansas City, Miss.: Sheed and Ward, 1988).

16. William David Ross, *The Right and the Good* (Oxford: Clarendon Press, 1930).

17. Karol Wojtyla, *The Acting Person*, trans. Osoba I. Czyn (Dordrecht, Holland/Boston: D. Reidel, 1979).

18. David C. Thomasma, "Hospital Ethics Committees and Hospital Policy," *Quality Review Bulletin* 7 (July 1985): 204–209.

19. Edmund D. Pellegrino, "Hospitals as Moral Agents: Some Notes on Institutional Ethics," in *Proceedings of the Third Annual Board of Trustees/Medical Staff Executive Committee Conference* (St. Joseph's Hospital, St. Paul, Minnesota March 26, 1977), pp. 10–27.

20. Richard M. Zaner, *Ethics and the Clinical Encounter* (Englewood Cliffs, N.J.: Prentice Hall, 1988), pp. 84–86.

21. From an unpublished manuscript by Andre Hellegers as quoted in Richard A. McCormick, *Health and Medicine in the Catholic Tradition* (New York: Crossroad, 1987), p. 41.

22. Edmund D. Pellegrino and David C. Thomasma, *For the Patient's Good: The Restoration of Beneficence in Health Care* (New York: Oxford University Press, 1988), p. 94.

23. Edmund D. Pellegrino, "Rationing Health Care: The Ethics of Medical Gatekeeping," *Journal of Contemporary Health Law and Policy* 2 (1986): 23–45.

24. Daniel Callahan, *What Kind of Life: The Limits of Medical Progress* (Washington, D.C.: Georgetown University Press, 1995).

25. Mark Siegler, "Treating the Jobless for Free: Do Doctors Have a Special Duty?" *Hastings Center Report* 3, no. 4 (1983): 12–14.

26. Alasdair MacIntyre, *After Virtue* (Notre Dame, Ind.: University of Notre Dame Press, 1981).

27. David C. Thomasma, "The Possibility of a Normative Medical Ethics," *Journal of Medicine and Philosophy* 5, no. 3 (1980): 249–259.

5

Religion and the Principles of Medical Ethics

The world today needs Christians who remain Christians.
Albert Camus, *Resistance, Rebellion, and Death*[1]

The Christian health professional is bound, like others, by the norms of philosophical medical ethics. From that source he or she derives principles, guidelines, rules, and codes that specify right and good actions and the criteria by which they may be judged. For the Christian, this is not, however, the whole of ethics. To be sure, the Christian perspective does not add another whole set of specific prescriptions; but the Christian ethic enjoins one overriding principle: love of God and neighbor. This creates special supererogatory obligations that might be options in another ethic. Thus, it is more than just a matter of holding certain beliefs that lead to specific behaviors. Religious ethics impels toward actions that oblige the person who holds the belief to act less selfishly in response to his or her own legitimate self-interests.

Most religions require some form or other of love of neighbor, of taking care of the community. The "Golden Rule" ethics, doing unto others as one would like done to oneself, can be found in most revealed religions and even in the "philosophical" religions. Jesus was a Jew who pulled his own insights out of the Jewish tradition.

CHRISTOCENTRIC HEALTH CARE ETHICS

The distinguishing factor of Christocentric ethics is the fact of revelation—a point that Frankena acknowledged in his classification of Christian ethics as agapeistic.[2] This difference does not yield precise indications, rules, or guidelines to determine what should be done in every given situation. Nor does it, of necessity, preclude the use of deontological or utilitarian principles in this or that decision. It requires only that any principle or ethical theory conform to the spirit of love and justice exemplified in the life, work, and teaching of Jesus Christ.

The Christian perspective therefore provides principles of discernment more than a code of rules for action. What it lacks in specificity, it gains in insight. It is a beacon and a compass that individual Christians and the Church must use to find the direction their faith requires them to follow. This is a task at once demanding and perilous. The call is to perfection—and the precise recipe for success is not available. Further, as times change and as new technological advances appear, the answer must continuously be reexamined and retested.

Christocentric ethics is therefore, in its deepest sense, "beyond" ethics. Romano Guardini puts it very well: "Once we restrict the word ethics to its modern specific sense of moral principles, it no longer accurately covers the Sermon on the Mount. What Jesus revealed there on the mountainside was no mere ethical code, but a whole new existence."[3] Guardini's point is that the Sermon on the Mount arises from an experience of ethics beyond philosophic insights alone. The important point is that the Sermon on the Mount most likely could not have been derived from a particular philosophical ethical theory.

This is not to dispose of ethics or law. Law impels us to limit self-interest for fear of punishment and thus assures an orderly society based on rights. Ethics impels us to limit self-interest as rational beings who recognize duties to others and thus assures a concerned and responsible social life. The mark of civilization is the extent to which ethics drives its laws, not the reverse. Religion in such a civilization impels us to limit self-interest because God asks us to do so out of love for him and his creatures and thus assures a caring society. This is something of what Guardini means when he says: "Only in love is genuine fulfillment of the ethical possible."[4]

Philosophical ethics can define the proper relationship between human beings, but not between God and humans, or between humans as God wants those relationships to be. A Christocentric ethic therefore does not repudiate philosophical ethics but transvalues its highest principles, justice and beneficence, into love and thereby carries them beyond the highest human aspirations.

There are, of course, specific moral principles and rules to guide adherents of different denominations. For Catholics, for example, these are found in the promulgations of the Moral Code for Catholic Hospitals, the pastoral letters of the bishops, the writings of the theologians, and the teachings of the popes. Similar guidance is given other religious health care institutions from the sponsoring religious bodies. But these sources are, all in their own way, the products of discernment—of the way the institutional Church reads Christ's call to love and justice in health care. There are numerous instances today in which such principles of discernment are needed to guide specific decisions and actions. These touch on some of the most important issues in health care today. Let us turn now to a brief examination of some selected aspects of contemporary health care ethics to see where the vectors of Christian discernment point.

THE RELIGIOUS PERSPECTIVE

Does religion offer a different and unique content for philosophical reflection that is not open to philosophy? If so, then religious medical ethics would differ qualitatively from philosophical and secular medical ethics. If not, then the religious character of bioethical reflections would be indistinguishable from a more secular medical ethics. Such reflections would differ only in degree rather than kind. Most likely the differences would be judged negatively, in philosophy's favor, since religious medical ethics would seem to accept more arguments from authority than philosophy would.

The subject matter of medical ethics does remain the same for both religious and secular medical ethics. The mode of analysis and the principles used, however, are different in some respects, the same in others. As we shall see in later chapters, arguments about duties and obligations to the poor, or arguments about euthanasia, may differ from one another regardless of the beliefs of the participants in the dialogue. Most religious persons, however, would claim that their faith itself informs their beliefs and their conduct. Hence the arguments advanced by them ought to reveal the character of their beliefs. The irony is that these arguments are often presented as having universal appeal. Where religious beliefs are solidified by secular power, this irony can also lead to tragedy. The problem is that to the extent that one's beliefs inform one's ethics and one's actions and the greater their appropriateness to the faith of the community to which one belongs, simultaneously there is a temptation to impose one's beliefs and moral code on others who do not share those beliefs. We must constantly be aware of the impact our training and beliefs have on our ways of thinking and acting so that we do not inadvertently impose these on others.

Indeed the opportunity for abuse is meliorated by secular pluralism. H. Tristram Engelhardt has claimed that a secular and philosophical medical ethics can transcend individual religious beliefs in a pluralistic society. As a consequence, he holds that philosophical medical ethics is superior for the development of public policy.[5] This, as the thrust of our whole effort in this book should indicate, is a dangerously impoverished notion of societal ethics.

THE LIMITATIONS OF CONTEMPORARY BIOMEDICAL ETHICS

It is a curious fact that professional philosophers, with one or two possible exceptions, took very little interest in medical ethics until about two decades ago. There are writings in abundance about medical ethics, to be sure, usually by physicians, but these frequently contained more exhortative than formally argued positions. Often rhetorical questions were asked about who should make decisions, how, and whether one was playing God. Few physicians twenty years ago had any formal philosophical training. Most often, too, their interest in the questions posed by advances in their discipline came from theological concerns. Questions appeared precisely because a religious training about the value of human life butted directly against possibilities and realities of modern medical practice.

Twenty-five years ago, however, the situation changed drastically. Professional philosophers began to take notice of the complex dilemmas created by the expansion of medical technological possibilities. They began to write about these issues[6] and then to assume teaching posts in medical schools under the aegis of programs on the humanities in medicine or human values and ethics.[7] In America, these philosophers brought with them the dominant mode of philosophizing, with its roots in analytic Anglo-American ethics.

This approach proved highly successful. It fitted the moral pluralism of our society. It argued from prima facie principles of beneficence, justice, and autonomy, all of which paralleled American social and political philosophy and culture. These thinkers were also intellectually credible and had sufficient rigor to be congenially disposed to the scientific milieu of medical education and practice.

As of this writing more than 100 of the nation's 125 medical schools teach medical ethics in some form or another. Topics in biomedical ethics are among the most popular in continuing medical education of physicians and other health professionals. Thousands of articles on medical ethics and the philosophy of medicine appear in the English language each year. Clinical journals now invariably have one or two papers on ethical questions and public policy in every issue. More than 100 "centers" of bioethics and medical ethics have appeared in the major countries of the world, the majority of these in North America. Professional ethicists are found in full-time positions in medical schools and hospital corporate structures. They assist as well in clinical consults and on hospital ethics committees.[8]

Ethics has begun to influence public policy beginning with the widespread influence of the President's Commission for the Study of Ethical Problems in Medicine and Biomedical and Behavioral Research. Since then federal and state legislators have argued about and written laws pertaining to definitions of death, anatomical gifts, the distribution and sale of organs for transplantation, abortion, and the care of defective newborns and are considering legislation on voluntary active euthanasia, limitations on care for the aged, the allocation of health care resources, the rationing by prospective payment plans, the creation of human research embryos, etc.

Finally, biomedical ethics is now one of the most popular subjects in all the media, in private and public discourse and in literature. Everywhere the "ethical" questions are being discussed as significant issues in everyday life, extending beyond biomedical ethics to business, the law, government, and international relations.

Much of this is commendable. Our age will probably be noted by historians as the age in which ethics was debated more freely and extensively than in any previous democratic society. To be sure, ethical issues were the preoccupation of philosophers, theologians, and the educated classes in past eras. But never have the issues been so widely discussed by the general public, never have they been so directly relevant to decisions the ordinary citizen must make. Some time or other most Americans face decisions about discontinuance of life support measures in terminally ill family members or seriously ill infants with multiple congenital defects; many may face amniocentesis and the possibility of abortion; some people may have to donate organs for transplants; and some may have to accept the reality of open-heart transplantation. The possibilities and the anxieties of medical technology ultimately will reflect into everyone's life.

Moreover, we are all becoming aware that we must be concerned about cost containment in health care. The conviction that our resources are limited leads us as a nation to rationing and allocation decisions that generate dilemmas of social ethics to which we cannot be indifferent. For ultimately what is at stake is the kind of society we want, or ought, to be. This decision seems on the surface to be a political one, but for most Americans it is also infused with religious values and commitments. This was all too painfully evident in the expansion and rapid collapse of the Health Care Reform debate of 1994. In our view, the administration's effort at reform uncovered too many beliefs and values that were held by Americans about their health care and that could not be papered over by public-relations programs or histrionics about cost escalation. The tragedy of a lack of health care for the uninsured and underinsured continues as a result, even though most Americans want equity for these persons as well.

After twenty-five years of biomedical ethics we find that there are some things that can be decided to the general satisfaction of most people. These are matters largely in the sphere of procedural ethics, that is to say, the ethics of the decision-making process that emphasizes the autonomy of patients and families and takes into account the heterogeneity of our moral-belief systems. This ethical process eschews the classical quest of normative ethics for universalizable norms of behavior that point to the right and the good and help define a good society. Indeed, given the clear indication that moral pluralism and the libertarian ethic are permanent features of American life, it is not an overstatement to say that normative ethics has largely been abandoned.

What alternatives are, then, open for those who persist in the feeling that procedural and analytical ethics are insufficient? What modes of ethics discourse are equal to the need so many persons have to do what is right although they disagree with the outcome of the analytical approach even when it is most rigorously followed? After all, there comes a time when balancing arguments becomes a futile exercise, since the case for contradictory actions seems so finely balanced that there is little to choose between the actions. We might conclude that this means that almost any choice would be morally defensible. Often this is the case, since the choices are not between obvious good and palpable evil but between two goods, both of which are to be desired. Others, however, would "feel" that one course is definitely wrong and bad and another right and good. How could these feelings be justified? Would they be simply the promptings of past religious training, conditioning by beliefs that are now seen as irrelevant to contemporary issues? Worse, would these feelings be dismissed as examples of the psychological need to control others, or the needless fretting of persons who take it upon themselves to be the conscience of society? Are the feelings that some things are wrong and others right derived from moral bigotry?

Moreover, there is the problem of motivation to do the right and the good. It is one thing to recognize a good argument for a particular course of action. It is another to be motivated to follow the conclusions of that argument.

Then there are those who dispose of all moral arguments as hair splitting or *post factum* rationalizations. These persons reject analytical ethics entirely. Many physicians, for example, take the analytical approach to be little more than a hubristic exercise in which some persons, self-appointed as "ethicists," make a living by telling other people what they ought to do.

Most telling of the limitations of analytical ethics is its failure to provide some ordering principles that cannot be trumped. The idea of prima facie principles such as beneficence, autonomy, and justice is extremely useful. But analytic ethics holds that it is the very nature of prima facie principles that they apply unless there are overriding reasons for setting them aside. One can then question what measure can be proposed that is sufficiently powerful enough to override a prima facie principle.

These limitations of the dominant analytical methodology of present-day biomedical ethics often lead people to take several alternative conceptual turns. These turns are to the intuitive, egotistic, or virtue theories of ethics. These too have their limitations.

All intuitive modes of doing ethics are variations of the moral-statement theories of Hume, Hutcheson, Smith, and Shaftsbury. They postulate a moral sense embedded in human consciousness that gives rise to the sentiment that a contemplated action is either right or wrong. But this leaves unresolved the central question—How do we decide between two individuals who arrive, by honest response to their own moral sentiments, at diametrically opposite positions? Are there good and bad moral sentiments embodied in different persons? Or is there a good moral sentiment in all? Is this sense taught, in which case would it be subject to the whims of society, or is it innate?

Virtue theories of ethics are regaining popularity after a lapse in the past two decades. They are the oldest theories of ethics, based in the notion of the good person, the one who habitually is disposed to make the right and the good decision. Such a person has learned, through practice of the virtues, to be virtuous. But the problem with virtue theories is that they involve circular reasoning. Virtue is what the good person has who habitually acts virtuously. But definitions of virtue vary, so that what is virtuous for one is vicious for another. Many of us can recall Buddhist monks in Vietnam setting themselves on fire to protest not only the war but also the involvement of the West in their culture. For them this was the highest virtuous act. Seeing this action on television was stupefying and horrendous for most Americans. How do we resolve these contradictions? How do we connect virtues with rights, duties, principles, and rules in ethics? Is there any connection at all between these modes of doing ethics?[9]

Variations of the virtue and moral sentiment theories are those based in process philosophy and in theories of discernment. Here again we are left with the problem of how to decide an issue when people of good will discern the right and good differently. Is one person evil, sick, disassembled? Do not all of these alternatives to principle-based ethics drive us to relativism and even to the destruction of ethics as a rational discipline?

There is another alternative that is not given much weight in philosophical circles. Understandably, this alternative is neglected by philosophical medical ethics, since it is religious and theological in foundation. A theological perspective is still important for many Americans. Many of the most irreconcilable differences in biomedical ethics derive from disagreements in religious points of view. As we mentioned in the first section of this chapter, this very disagreement leads some thinkers, such as Engelhardt, to reject a religious basis for medical ethics in favor of a secular, libertarian one.

The problem for religious ethics is that it relies for its foundations on an externally derived given. This may be revealed truth or some insight of the religion's founder, such as Buddha's insight of the principle of constant change. How does this given differ from the "moral sense" just described, or from Kant's "good will"? From Engelhardt's point of view, rationality or logic is the common denominator for sorting out all these foundational claims that legitimate religious ethical theories. One might counter that there is something transcendent that unites all religious viewpoints. But once again, is it not logic that searches out this fundament among them?

Notwithstanding this problem, we believe the religious perspective deserves a hearing. It has much to offer to believers and nonbelievers, if it is not taken as a morally superior position or a monochromatic one. In this way it can complement and supplement the important contribution analytical ethics has already made to the advances of biomedical ethical thinking in our day.

THE CONTENT

Religious and secular medical ethics often concern the same issues and questions. But a secular medical ethics may miss some of the important insights that religious belief brings to the entire enterprise of medicine and health care. Engelhardt's secular medical ethics, for example, would lay the basis for a minimalist social policy that could miss the importance of many other features of the human community. In fact, his own development of the primacy of the principle of autonomy over the importance of the role of the community reflects this bias.[10]

Contrast his secular view with that of Bernard Häring, who notes: "The unfolding of life and its protection, health and healing, death and dying, are all decisive focal points for social responsibility. Bioethics cannot be separated from the broader task of Christians to join hands for the building up of a healthier world."[11]

That a secular view may neglect important insights for medical ethics, public policy, and the nature of medicine is a basic premise of this book. To be sure, there are other viewpoints than Engelhardt's that would provide a richer and more accurate articulation of the nature of the community. These insights are not hidden to philosophical reflection. Believers of revealed religion, however, hold certain insights to be more important than do philosophy and other secular disciplines, such as medical sociology and medical anthropology. These disciplines may, in fact, acknowledge the importance of a transcendent element in sickness and healing, of the value of human life, and so on. But they do not build their arguments on the *primacy* of such insights.

Further, as St. Thomas Aquinas argued about theology itself, without revealed religious beliefs, only a few human beings would arrive at important conclusions and only after a long period of time, with a great mixture of error.[12] Considering the human propensity for error in any case, the claim of a religious medical ethics is that it may be based on principles that guide all human affairs from the point of view of the Creator of such affairs. This is an extrahuman perspective, one that critiques all human enterprises and subjects them to a layer of analysis not existent in secular medical ethics.

In this respect, St. Thomas notes that what revealed religion provides to secular insights is the notion that there is an end to human life beyond this world. This end should propel our thinking and acting: "Above all because God destines us for an end beyond the grasp of reason. . . . Now we have to recognize an end before we can stretch out and exert ourselves for it."[13]

The calling to a task to build the earth and to live life in the spirit of altruism and charity does make a difference in the ways in which persons will analyze their own roles in the tasks of medicine. It also leads to a difference in analysis of ethical issues, as subsequent chapters will show.

MOTIVATION

A religious medical ethics provides a reason to be moral. Philosophers themselves have argued at great length about the ultimate motive to be moral. Reason and habit (virtue) can be motivations to be moral, but they are originally supplied by the community whose responsibility it is to teach the young such virtues. Thus, motivation is circular. We are motivated to be moral by training supplied by the community that finds it good to be moral.

Essentially the religious reason to be moral is to please God, who has told us to be good and has revealed what it means to be good as a creature. It is not only a community's perception of the good that impels morality. The ultimate good of human beings is defined in a religious medical ethics as a transcendent good, a good beyond the individual, beyond self-interest. This point should be taken with caution. Often believers hold that God pours out infinite love for human beings and that imitating God means that one should never focus on oneself. Selfishness is abjured.[14] This point of view is so directly opposed to the libertarian that those who follow a religious ethics do not just disagree with thinkers such as Engelhardt. They are offended by him. A response by Stanley Hauerwas to Engelhardt at an annual meeting of the Society for Health and Human Values pointed out this clash with intense vigor, for Hauerwas holds that Engelhardt's vision of the community and human meaning is fatally flawed and directly opposed to a true vision of the meaning of human existence.[15]

But this can be said in Engelhardt's favor: autonomy and self-determination are important features of any theory of human existence, religious or otherwise. It would be unhealthy to hold that persons must give up their own self-interest in helping others. Otherwise they would become victims of other people's agendas. On the positive side, there is an obligation to protect one's own life, well-being, family, and even goods.

Instead, what is at stake is where to put the emphasis. Secular medical ethics has placed it squarely on autonomy because it meshes so clearly with the political and social goals of the United States. It can be derived from our political philosophy and the history of successive civil-rights movements. And finally, autonomy and rights thinking can propose clearly understood behaviors for others. If I have a right or an entitlement, others have duties to me.

Religious medical ethics puts the emphasis on the community, on the good of others in that community. It recognizes the grounding of autonomy in the dignity of human persons. But it does place it on a relative scale second to beneficence, acting for the good of others.[16] The whole point of having freedom is not license but rather the ability to do what one ought to do.

Religion also closes the moral gap between cognition of the right and good and doing the right and good thing. It supplies the motivation to act for the good of others, a motivation that philosophical methodology alone cannot supply. Recall that Socrates thought that knowledge of the good would automatically lead to acting on the basis of the good. St. Paul, though, realized that we often act otherwise than our convictions: "I can will what is right, but I cannot do it. For I do not do the good I want, but the evil I do not want is what I do."[17] We know, especially since the time of Freud, that there is a dark side to human nature that impedes the translation of the intellectually conceived good to a morally good action.

It is not easy to implement our convictions. In this instance, religious medical ethics impels the spirit toward sacrifice and courage. Once again it should be stressed that if the conviction happens to be wrong, a religious ethics can quickly create a religious zealot or religious bigot. Witness some televangelists.

Frankly, many people reject a religious ethics for very sound reasons. They are actually rejecting bigotry and condemnatory features that too often have accompanied religion in its stormy history. Such negative influence creates a bad name for religion and consequently the valuable insights it can offer in the resolution of thorny dilemmas we face. It is often said that hard cases make bad law. Comparably bad religious thinking and actions create bad ethics.

ORDERING PRINCIPLE

Religion also provides an ordering principle whereby conflicts among goods, principles, and moral sentiments can be resolved. In the Jewish tradition, the Law, the prophets, life as a people, the remnant of the community—all play a role in casuistic resolutions of conflicts. In Christian resolutions, charity is the ordering principle, and agapeistic ethics must predominate.[18] One balances charitable justice (justice as the voice of love), beneficence, self-interest, and other principles by a call to perfection. The individual facing the dilemma adds an extra layer of analysis to the philosophical by asking what God wants him or her to do in this situation. From a Christian perspective, the community is as important as the individual. Autonomy is constrained and is not the primary principle of medical ethics, as we have already discussed.

With a religious point of view, there are problems that must be recognized. These do not vitiate that point of view; rather they demonstrate the inability of some persons to be faithful to what they preach, or even to understand the full impact of that teaching. For example:

1) There is conflict on important issues between and within different belief systems. Abortion is one example. Some Jews and Christians find it abhorrent. Others do not. Hence, appeals to religious

principles to delineate conflicts with secular society may be charged with inconsistency and thus easily disposed of. Even though the Catholic Church condemns abortion, persons citing themselves as Catholics are statistically as likely to obtain an abortion as any other group of Americans.[19] Findings such as these cast serious doubts on the strength or quality of religious belief as an influence on ethics.

2) Law and morality conflict in our society as well. Although abortion is legal, many hold it to be immoral. Although euthanasia is illegal, many hold it to be moral. Consider the case of Dr. Kevorkian in Michigan, a pathologist who invented the "death machine," a device whereby persons, by pressing a button or inhaling a lethal gas, can kill themselves. Mrs. Janet Adkins from Portland, Oregon, was selected by "Dr. Death," as he has come to be called, for the first try. The device worked, and she died, asking him to tell her story.[20]

In the fallout about this case it quickly became clear that both the law and society must become more specific about the difference between assisted suicide, active euthanasia, and murder. Further, even if there is a difference, what does this imply for public policy? At least an additional twenty-one persons have been helped by Dr. Kevorkian since, while the public debate continues. Some religious thinkers wonder whether taking responsibility for our technology might mean that we should open the door to death just as we can often close it.[21] Others roundly condemn Dr. Death's action as a violation of the rule against killing.

3) Institutional conflicts also occur. One distressing example of this is the cutthroat competition for patient care dollars among some religiously sponsored hospitals in large cities. Competition rather than cooperation drives the quest for institutional survival. In this environment, one wonders how a religious perspective contributes to building up the community through social justice when the opposite seems to be the case within the religious community itself! The local ordinaries are now effecting a policy that requires their approval for merges between Catholic and other health care institutions so that the Catholic identity in health care may not be lost to the need to compete.

4) There are also problems at the edge of the foundations of ethics itself. Perhaps the most telling is the current movement grounding ethics in biology. On the one hand, sociobiologists such as Edward O. Wilson argue very strenuously that ethical behaviors, for example

altruism, are merely biological inducements, programs in the very makeup of DNA. On the other hand, there are theorists, particularly those philosophers of biology who seem to have rediscovered evolutionary thought, who hold that Darwinism is directly opposed to religious thought and that the former offers a far more cogent theory of development than the latter. Thus William Provine of Cornell University argues that one must choose either Darwin or God when examining the implications of evolutionary biology. Provine suggests that one must check one's brains at the church house door if one accepts evolutionary biology: "The frequently-made assertion that modern biology and the assumptions of the Judeo-Christian tradition are fully compatible is false."[22] His argument is that evolution is not a purposive activity. Thus, evolutionary theory counters a fundamental belief not only of religious persons but of most persons in Western civilization.

Provine makes two assumptions that are highly problematic, however. The first is that modern science implies that the world is composed of strictly mechanistic principles. The second is that modern science implies that there are no inherently moral or ethical laws, no absolute guiding principles for society. He concludes that "we humans are just complex machines without free will that have been poorly programmed for moral behavior."[23] This is a contemporary statement as naive as La Mettrie's simplistic Cartesian mechanism of the eighteenth century and is inconsistent with philosophy as well as science.[24]

MEDICINE'S CONTRIBUTION TO RELIGIOUS ETHICS

Our emphasis has by design been on the way the religious and theological perspective may enrich and enhance medical ethics. It must not be forgotten that medicine can have a positive influence on religions and theology, too. There are several ways in which this can come about.

First of all, medicine supplies the factual clinical and scientific data upon which coherent speculative thought must be based. Many ethical debates are futile and divisive because they begin from insecure or even erroneous scientific data.[25] Despite admonitions to the contrary from the more sophisticated practitioners of other disciplines, science and theology still do not enjoy a sufficiently penetrating relationship with each other.[26] As a result, what has always been a false dichotomy between faith and scientific reason is propagated further. Given the powerful influence of science on culture and medicine, to neglect this dialogue is to hamper theological discourse and diminish its intellectual credibility.[27]

Second, medicine is a source for the phenomenological particularities that can give verisimilitude and credibility to biomedical ethical discourse, whether it is predominantly philosophical or theological. This happens when the theologian is immersed in the experiences of suffering; in the actualities of disease, illness, and death; and in the urgency, complexity, and emotional milieu within which concrete decisions must be made. If perchance the theologian, as those in clinical medicine deem advisable, observes actual decision making, or takes part in discussions of concrete cases, or acts as a bioethics consultant in the clinical setting, the relationships of abstract deduced principles to concrete clinical situations will be more sensitively appreciated. There is no doubt that the theologian must retain a certain distance from day-to-day decision making, but occasional immersion in those decisions will counter the tendency to oversimplify or to ignore the all-encompassing reality, the professional and human dimensions, that shape and nuance actual decision making and moral choice.

Third, medicine provides a rich source of feedback for the reality testing of religious thinking and theological principles as well as of ecclesial regulation of the relation of technology to human affairs. This is not to suggest that the difficulty of adherence to theological principles might be an excuse for ignoring them. Rather it does suggest that actual experience in implementing these principles may uncover neglected nuances about the existential situation. This could lead to a more critical reexamination of theological positions. In essence what seems requisite is a continuing dialogue between theological speculation and clinical experience.

CONCLUSION

The general scope of a religious medical ethics embraces another layer of critical insight against which human reason is judged. That layer arises from a calling beyond this life that relativizes (but does not diminish) all other absolutes posed by secular systems of thought. Our endeavor will show how a religious medical ethics brings an added dimension of analysis to the debates about actions that disvalue human life.

NOTES

1. Albert Camus, *Resistance, Rebellion, and Death* (New York: Alfred Knopf, 1961), p. 70.

2. William Frankena, *Ethics,* 2d ed. (Englewood Cliffs, N.J.: Prentice-Hall, 1973).

3. Romano Guardini, *The Lord* (Chicago: Henry Regnery, 1954), p. 79.

4. Guardini, *The Lord,* p. 84. It has been pointed out that, for Kant, what is praiseworthy in ethics is that which is done in spite of inclination. In theory, for Kant, if we act well toward others out of love and compassion for them, our actions are less praiseworthy than if they were done with no such inclination.

5. H. Tristram Engelhardt, Jr., "Philosophical Medical Ethics," in *Health/Medicine and the Faith Traditions: An Enquiry into Religion and Medicine,* ed. Martin E. Marty and Kenneth L. Vaux (Philadelphia: Fortress Press, 1982).

6. Two scholarly initiatives encouraged this interest: The first was the creation of the *Journal of Medicine and Philosophy* within the Society for Health and Human Values; the second was the development of a series entitled Philosophy and Medicine by D. Reidel/Kluwer Academic Publishers under the editorship of H. Tristram Engelhardt, Jr., and Stuart Spicker, both philosophers.

7. Thomas K. McElhinney and Edmund D. Pellegrino, *Teaching Ethics, the Humanities, and Human Values in Medical Schools: A Ten Year Overview* (Washington, D.C.: Society for Health and Human Values, 1982).

8. It is good to be cautious about all this activity for fear of "protesting too much." While all this ethical activity may demonstrate a solidly value-oriented state of affairs, it may also demonstrate a declining state of affairs in which greed and self-interest prevail, the interest in ethics being nothing but a ruse to mask the decline.

9. See Edmund D. Pellegrino and David C. Thomasma, *The Virtues in Medical Practice* (New York: Oxford University Press, 1993); and *The Christian Virtues in Medicine* (Washington, D.C.: Georgetown University Press, 1995).

10. H. Tristram Engelhardt, Jr., *The Foundations of Bioethics* (New York: Oxford University Press, 1986).

11. Bernard Häring, *Free and Faithful in Christ: Moral Theology for Clergy and Laity,* vol. 3 (New York: Crossroad, 1981), p. 3.

12. St. Thomas Aquinas, *Summa Theologiae,* vol. 1, trans. Thomas Gilby (New York: McGraw-Hill/Blackfriars, 1964), Ia-I, art. 1, reply, pp.6–9.

13. Aquinas, *Summa Theologiae,* Vol. 1, p. 7.

14. Stephen Post, "The Inadequacy of Selflessness: God's Suffering and the Theory of Love," *Journal of the American Academy of Religion* 56, no. 2 (1988): 213–228.

15. Stanley Hauerwas, "Response to Engelhardt's *The Foundations of Bioethics,*" Annual Meeting, Society for Health and Human Values, (New Orleans, November 1987).

16. See our discussion of the strengths and weaknesses of autonomy-based and beneficence-based ethics in Edmund D. Pellegrino and David C. Thomasma, *For the Patient's Good: The Restoration of Beneficence in Health Care* (New York: Oxford University Press, 1988), pp. 11–36.

17. Romans 7:18–19, in *Holy Bible: Revised Standard Version* (New York: Thomas Nelson, 1972).

18. Edmund D. Pellegrino, "Agape and Ethics: Some Reflections on Medical Morals from a Catholic Christian Perspective," in *Catholic Perspectives on Medical Morals*, ed. Edmund D. Pellegrino, John P. Langan, and John C. Harvey (Dordrecht, Holland/Boston: Kluwer Academic Publishers, 1989), pp. 277–300.

19. James Kelly, "Catholic Abortion Rates and the Abortion Controversy," *America* 160, no. 4 (1989): 82–85.

20. Timothy Egan, "As Memory and Music Faded, Alzheimer Patient Met Death," *New York Times* (June 7, 1990): A1, D22.

21. Kenneth Vaux, "If We Can Bar the Door to Death, Can We Also Open It?" *Chicago Tribune* (February 10, 1988): A23.

22. William Provine, "Evolution and the Foundation of Ethics," *MBL Science* 3, no. 1 (1988): 25–29.

23. Provine, "Evolution and the Foundation of Ethics," p. 29.

24. Julien Offray de La Mettrie, *L'homme machine*, 1748.

25. William A. Wallace, "Nature and Human Nature as the Norm in Medical Ethics," in *Catholic Perspectives*, ed. Pellegrino, Langan, and Harvey, pp. 23–54.

26. Edmund D. Pellegrino, "The Humanities in Medical Education: Entering the Post–Evangelical Era," *Theoretical Medicine* 5, no. 3 (1984): 254–266.

27. Edmund D. Pellegrino, "Science and Theology, from a Medical Perspective," *Linacre Quarterly* 57, no. 4 (1990): 19–35.

6

Medicine as a Calling

Even in the most secular ethic, the idea of a profession carries within it a sense of special commitment. On naturalistic grounds alone the obligation to pursue something beyond self-interest has long been identified as a characteristic of the learned professions. While medicine itself cannot be said to be a religion according to our definition, for some, such as the doctor in Albert Camus's *The Plague*, it functions as a substitute.[1] In this chapter we will examine the way a religious, and explicitly a Christian, perspective enriches and expands the idea of a profession.

Religious belief transforms a profession into a vocation and distances both from an occupation. A vocation is a call to a way of life defined not solely by the set of activities that constitute a career or by even the pursuit of an ethical occupation within constraints that might normally define a profession. A vocation to the Christian life entails the metamorphosis of even the most mundane activity to the level of a grace, a way of giving witness to the gospel message in every activity, no matter how mundane or technical it may be.

The key question we must address is this: what is the difference in obligations between an occupation, a profession, and a vocation or calling?

INTRODUCTION

The idea of a profession has long centered on the notion that certain activities are moral enterprises calling for altruistic service and some effacement of self-interest. When these moral aspirations are highly developed, professions become vocations; when they are downgraded, professions become careers. The direction of these shifts is of the utmost importance in society.

Today, the shift is in the direction of self-interest. There is a growing loss of faith in the idea that any group can be dedicated to other than self-interest. What is even more significant is the deeper current of drift in the moral philosophy of the professions, a shift in paradigms that would justify downgrading their moral commitments.

Is this moral drift reversible? Should it be reversed? What are the philosophical underpinnings of professional morality? This chapter offers some reflections on the current direction of professional morality, its causation and effects, and on the desirability of a more explicit moral philosophy of the professions.

While the issues are conceptual, their practical consequences are enormous. We are a society ever more dependent on the uses of specialized knowledge. The professional purveyors of that knowledge make crucial decisions that affect all of us. Ultimately, we are dependent on the moral character of the decisions and their authors. The moral defections of doctors, lawyers, corporate executives, scientists, engineers, and even ministers constitute a grave danger in a technological and industrialized society.

There is clear evidence of a moral drift in the notion of a profession in such morally repugnant events as Auschwitz, Watergate, Bhopal, insider trading, the Iran debacle, Medicaid frauds, falsification of research, and defense contract cheating.[2] It is distressing in each instance to see the failure of the "professionals" to admit to or even recognize their lapses as moral lapses. Perhaps more distressing still is the public apathy about, and even the rational justification of, these moral lapses. Clearly, some radical shift in our moral perspective of what constitutes a profession is taking place in our time.

Each generation holds stewardship over the traditions it receives, and is accountable for the transformation in those traditions it effects and transmits to its successors. Our generation, therefore, has a serious obligation to examine its tradition on professions—what of it is to be retained, what discarded, and what added. Neither a complete restoration of the ancient edifice nor its demolition is morally defensible. The real challenge is to reconstruct an idea of professional morality responsive to the need for change without sacrificing the distinctive elements that set professions off from other human activities.

Medicine is a paradigm of the descent from vocation to career. It has the longest history of explicit ethical commitment. Its moral perspectives have undergone more profound transformation in the last twenty years than in all of its previous history. Finally, it is a helping profession, one that purports to fill a fundamental human need. For this reason it is quintessentially a moral enterprise.

Medicine epitomizes the dilemmas faced by all the other helping professions. Law aims to meet the need for justice, ministry for salvation, and education for knowledge. Like medicine, each is a moral enterprise because each requires a vulnerable person to trust in the competence and goodwill of someone who professes to help. Each of these professions involves a relationship morally grounded in the needs of wounded or afflicted humanity.

We will limit our considerations to professional morality—the sum of obligations that arise out of the special nature of the activity in which a profession engages. This is, in a formal sense, the internal morality of the profession. There are also innumerable concrete medical moral issues—for example, euthanasia, gene therapy, withdrawing life support, allocation of scarce resources, etc. A whole panoply of new ethical issues has entranced the public and the profession alike in recent years. These are of obvious importance. But what is fundamental to all of them is the morality of the physician-patient relationship, that component of medical ethics that comprises professional morality. It is the descent and reascent of moral integrity in professional ethics that will be our main focus.

THE TRADITION AND ITS MUTATIONS

The received professional ethics of a quarter-century ago was a compound of the ethics of the Oath and the deontological books of the Hippocratic corpus, modulated by Judaeo-Christian solicitude for the sick and reinforced in Anglo-American culture by the obligations owed by a gentlemanly class to the less fortunate members of a society.[3] This is the combination that constitutes the Medical Ethics of Thomas Percival, published in 1803 and subsumed almost verbatim into the first code of ethics of the American Medical Association in 1848.[4] Though it has been modified and drastically abbreviated, the ethos of the original A.M.A. code has constituted the tradition of medical ethics in our century.

That tradition rested on the notion of a beneficent, paternalistic "brotherhood" dedicated to a set of self-imposed moral obligations governing their relationships with the sick and with fellow physicians.[5] It enjoined beneficence, confidentiality, a life of "purity and holiness"; it forbade abortion, all forms of "mischief," and sexual relationships with patients or their families. There was no place for the patient's view of his own interests in making clinical decisions. The physician automatically enjoyed both moral and technical authority over the patient's welfare. No allowance was made for the social ethics of medicine or for the ethical obligations of other health professionals or families. Central to the whole tradition was the ideal of the profession as a select body dedicated primarily to the service of others rather than to self-interest.

Whatever its merits or demerits, this tradition was honored by the best physicians of ages past. Those who violated or ignored its precepts were moral pariahs, unworthy of membership in the profession. Many physicians, to be sure, did fail to live up to this ethic, and many even flaunted it. But when they did so, they were recognized as morally delinquent. Never were their actions legitimated or defended as morally acceptable alternatives.

Today, however, almost every precept of the traditional ethical canon is being questioned in principle. The very ideal of a noble calling is branded as elitist. The relationships of physician and patient are interpreted by some as more akin to a legal contract than a moral covenant; others argue for a commodity transaction or an exercise in applied biology. Abortions are now legal. Confidentiality can be violated in certain circumstances. Patient autonomy now overrides the physician's paternalism. Physician self-interest is exploited to limit costs in managed health systems. Some psychiatrists argue that sexual relations with patients are part of a therapeutic regimen. Others defend assisted suicide, and even direct and indirect euthanasia.

What is most significant in all of this is the challenge to the ideal of a profession as a group within society dedicated to a special way of life—a life of service in which self-interest yields to altruism. To practice medicine was tantamount to a vocation in the religious sense—even for those without formal religious ties. Medicine as a means of livelihood, prestige, power, and preferments—as a career—was secondary to medicine as a calling. But now increasing numbers of physicians—young and old—have abandoned the idea of medicine as a profession and a vocation. To them such ideals are untenable in today's sociocultural milieu.

Where formerly there was a "common devotion" to an ideal, there is today confusion, doubt, dissent, and depression.[6] The future of medical ethics is itself in doubt as a result. One of the most frequent questions from conscientious physicians is, "What is a good person to do?" They see the moral moorings of the profession loosening and as yet no clear sign of what will take their place.

At the heart of this moral confusion lies a loss of faith in the viability of the ancient ideal of a profession. The conviction is growing that medicine (and law or ministry) is not essentially different from business or its occupations. Why, then, should the professions be held to a standard of altruism not required of others? The erosion of moral standards in business, politics, and government now seems an acceptable reality to increasing numbers of people. Are not the inherited ideals of the professions simply unworkable in today's moral climate?

Many seriously doubt that a reconstruction of the idea of a profession is possible and that, as a consequence, there is a future for professional ethics. Fewer religious people subscribe to the ideal of a vocation. The exigencies of modern life seem too powerful to be resisted even with the help of a faith commitment.

Any response to these questions must turn first to the forces producing such profound changes in so short a time. These forces have exposed defects in some parts of the tradition and distorted others dangerously. Separating defect from distortion is difficult but not impossible, provided some ordering principles are in hand to structure the sorting process.

GENESIS OF THE MUTATIONS

First among those forces is the rise of participatory democracy. Benign authoritarianism is no longer acceptable, nor are the fraternal protectionism and the presumption of privilege and prerogative that constituted some of the less admirable traits of the established professionals.

Coupled to participatory democracy is public education. The inner workings of the professions are now subjects of wide popular interest. Novels, television programs, newspaper stories, and soap operas revel in the triumphs and failings of professional life. The professions have been demystified. Cynicism has grown as the difficulties and dilemmas of professional life are exposed to public view.

Mistrust of the whole profession is fueled by periodic revelations of unethical physician misbehavior, from its grossest example in the Nazi doctors to the lesser but more frequent lapses in Medicaid fraud, insensitivity to the care for the poor, or conspicuous consumerism.[7]

No less damaging has been the repeated resistance of the organized profession in the last few decades to reforms in the health care delivery system.

Simultaneously the public has become aware of the ubiquity and complexity of the genuine moral dilemmas associated with modern medical care. Cases such as those of Karen Quinlan, Baby Doe and Baby Fae, Bouvia, Whitehead, Cruzan, and others have made it obvious that physicians have had to make moral choices that sooner or later touched on everyone's life.[8]

Perhaps the most significant factor of all is the growth of moral diversity in American life. Moral pluralism had incubated for a long time in American society, but in the late sixties it became explicit. The presumption of a homogeneous value system based in the Judaeo-Christian ethic was seriously challenged. Doctor and patient could no longer assume consensus on the most fundamental questions about human life, its meaning, purpose, and worth. Instead of a community bound together by shared values, moral individualism has become the rule.

The deeper consequences of moral pluralism were several. For one thing, patients and doctors increasingly turned to the courts to resolve moral disputes. Legal decisions have taken on moral force. For another, patient autonomy is supplanting beneficence as the dominant principle in medical ethics. Finally, moral neutrality and relativism became dominant theories in ethics. Ethics itself has lost much of its classical normative thrust and is confined by many solely to conceptual analysis.

With the loss of faith in an objective order of morality, economics, law, and social custom have come to be the ultimate sources of morality in the minds of many physicians, patients, and policy makers. The deep and often irreconcilable differences in fundamental precepts have shifted the locus of ethical discourse from substance to procedure.

The convergence of these forces has reduced the number of moral precepts held in common by physicians. The profession is now divided on several fronts—first, on what constitutes a profession, second, on the specific moral issues of abortion, voluntary euthanasia, and reproductive technologies, and, third, on the nature of the physician-patient relationship.

There is no likelihood that the substantive changes brought about by sociocultural forces will be reversed completely. Nor it is desirable that this happen. Some are morally salubrious, e.g., the trend to autonomy, to patient participation, and to explicit public dialogue about medical issues; the courses in biomedical ethics; the regularization of procedures for decision making; the new emphasis on the social obligation of physicians; and the recommendations of the President's Commission for the Study of Ethical Problems in Medicine and Biomedical and Behavioral Research.

In fact, the most significant changes have remedied defects or omissions in traditional medical ethics. The result is a more open, more adult, and mutually more responsible physician-patient relationship. To this extent, changes in the tradition enhance, rather than detract from, the moral quality of medical transactions.

Gratifying as some of the recent changes may be, others are disturbing indeed. These threaten the most precious element in the older tradition—the idea of altruistic service as a moral obligation intrinsic to certain kinds of human activity. If there is to be a reversal of the downward moral drift in the profession, we must rethink the concept of a profession—and the moral obligations that flow from it.

THE INTERNAL MORALITY OF THE PROFESSIONS

What is it that distinguishes certain activities as true professions? How do they differ in kind from all the other occupations that claim this title? Generally the answer has been given in the sociological rather than the philosophical literature. The distinction has usually been based on the attributes of a profession, its social functions, or its sociohistorical context.

To define a profession by its attributes is to beg the question of what a profession is. It is simply to annotate those attributes one presupposes to be professional and those that are not. By the usual roster of attributes, many activities, from playing football to hairdressing and selling used cars, might qualify.[9]

Definition by function, as in the definitive studies of Talcott Parsons, is conceptually more substantial.[10] Though sociologically inspired, Parsons's definitions are normative in spirit and argue for certain moral obligations, such as competence and effacement of self-interest, because they are essential to performance of the social functions of medicine. This view corresponds in some degree to the view we espouse later in this chapter.

Pernick and others hold that there is no fixed definition of a profession. Rather, Pernick argues: "professionalism is an instrumental value, a changing tool for solving changing problems rather than a fixed set of traditional solutions."[11]

With the exception possibly of Parsons's view, none of these definitions provides a substantial foundation for the moral obligations of the professional. Each would, in its own way, accommodate the moral drift that is our central concern here.

Against these views we contend that there is something fixed and unchangeable in the idea of a profession. In the specific case of medicine, it is the nature of illness, the act of profession, and the nature of the medical act. One of us has argued this thesis elsewhere.[12] For this purpose, we isolate and define four phenomenological characteristics of a profession, more specifically, of the helping professions. The moral character of medicine as a profession is grounded in these characteristics.

The four features that are fundamental to a true profession are 1) the nature of the human needs it addresses, 2) the vulnerable state of those it serves, 3) the expectations of trust it generates, and 4) the social contract it implies. Taken together, these features set the traditional ideal of a profession apart from other occupations that lay claim to the title. These are characteristics in any healing and helping relationship. They cut across cultures, geographic locations, and historical epochs because they are grounded in experiences common to all humanity. That some professions use these phenomena to their own advantage or otherwise distort them does not destroy their validity.[13]

To begin with, the needs with which the helping professions deal are needs most closely associated with being human. Health, knowledge, salvation, and justice are essential to our fulfillment as human persons. When we have lost them, our humanity itself is wounded. We remain persons, but impaired in our capacities to live fully as persons. We cannot enjoy the other dimensions of our lives. For this reason, the professions that help us regain our wounded humanity—medicine, law, and ministry—have a special place in society.

To lack health, for example, imposes limitations that the lack of most other things does not. When we are ill, as we have shown, we cannot pursue fully any of our other goals and aspirations. Our whole life's agenda must be held in abeyance until our illness is either cured, contained, or palliated. To heal requires the physician not only to treat an organ and a symptom but to enter the private world of the self. Even if the illness is beyond science or art, the physician is expected to help the patient manage the experience of illness.

In order that the physician may heal, the patient permits the physician certain freedoms not ordinarily accorded to strangers—freedom to delve into the most private experiences and thoughts, to invade the privacy of the body and the relationships with others. In different ways, this is true of the lawyer and the minister as well. It is not true of most other occupations. The banker, for example, may enter one intimate part of our life but not the whole of it as is necessary for the physician, lawyer, or minister.

Second, the existential state in which we consult these professionals is one of necessity and vulnerability. When we consult them, we have already realized that we can no longer cope with our afflicted state. We recognize we must call for help. We make a conscious decision to become a patient, a client, or a penitent. We enter a new state of dependency, anxiety, fear, pain, and disability. We are eminently vulnerable and eminently exploitable. We must seek out the physician's, lawyer's, or minister's help in a relationship that is unequal. The power to help, harm, or deceive rests with the professional. We must heal ourselves, too, but we need help to show us the way.

Third, no matter how much we have labored to achieve informed consent, to write a contract for what we expect will be done, or to seek consultation with others, we cannot escape the need to trust the practitioner. Ultimately, in the operating room, in the consulting room, in the court or the confessional, there comes a moment of trust when things can go well or ill. No contract can anticipate the decisions that the moment will require. Then it is the character of the professional and his or her willingness to place our welfare first that we must depend upon.

The patient has a moral claim on the physician to act in the patient's interest, even to the suppression of some self-interest in the patient's behalf. This expectation is grounded in the doctor's "profession," the offer to help, to put professional knowledge to use as the patient's advocate. The doctor's profession is a declaration in public and private that he or she can be trusted not to exploit the patient's vulnerability in any way. This promise is given publicly at the time of graduation when the physician declares to all present—and to all future patients—a commitment to fidelity to the promise of help. The same profession is made privately every time the physician offers to help or heal a sick person.

A fourth feature of the internal morality of a profession is the social contract it implies. Professions are granted the responsible use of certain privileges, e.g., wide discretionary space within which to decide and act, the rights of confidentiality, self-regulation, the establishment of standards of admission, accreditation, etc. These privileges are granted not primarily for the benefit of the profession but because they are essential to the profession's performance of certain functions essential to a civilized and healthy society. In a sense the professions are "ordained"—empowered to perform their specific functions and allowed the freedom necessary to do so.

This is especially the case in medicine. Medical knowledge is not proprietary. Society permits human experimentation, the dissection and autopsy of human bodies, the entry of neophytes into the actual care of patients, the free exchange of medical techniques and knowledge between societies—all because these are necessary for the effective training of the next generation of physicians. Such privileges cannot be construed as rights purchased by tuition payments. Nor can the knowledge derived from socially conferred privileges be used primarily as the means of personal and private profit or livelihood.

These four features of the relationship with a professional differ from an ordinary commodity transaction or a contract in the marketplace. In a genuine profession there is the expectation of beneficence, not simply nonmaleficence. The degree of beneficence expected goes beyond what is ordinarily required in our society. It entails doing good even at some personal sacrifice or risk. The physician who treats patients with contagious disease, the lawyer who defends the political prisoner, the criminal, or the poor, the priest who endangers his life to administer the rites of the dying, or the minister who counsels the sociopath and the paranoid—all respond to the obligation of compassion and effacement of self-interest built into the internal morality of a helping profession.

Some of the features of a profession we have enumerated bear a resemblance to Parsons's analyses of the same question. He places emphasis on the vulnerability of the sick person, the lack of power, and the dependence on the physician's knowledge. From these Parsons argues that the physician's role requires him or her to serve the patient's interests and prevent exploitation. To enable the physician to achieve these functional ends, society grants certain privileges—self-regulations, a fee structure, accreditation, freedom of decision, etc. The patient has a role too—to facilitate the physician's effort to heal him or her.

Parsons's analysis grounds the physician's obligations in social role and social utility—in the necessity to solve the problem of physician and patient facing illness. The purpose of their relationship is to reduce disability in society. The obligations of the profession are role norms, created by the professions to facilitate performance of their social functions.

The difficulty with this view is that the social function of medicine need not be defined in terms of the patient's interests. Medicine in Nazi Germany became the functional instrument of genocide; psychiatry in Soviet Russia was an instrument of political repression. Peter Frank's "Medical Police" used medicine as the instrument for securing economic productivity or military service.

Parsons justifies beneficence on the basis of the need to preserve the social system. When that system is best served by some other function, beneficence would have to yield. This is directly contrary to the central thrust of the traditional ethic of medicine, which—for the individual physician—makes the patient's interest primary, to be compromised only in the most extreme circumstances.

Parenthetically, on this point, Freidson's account seems closer to the one we are espousing.[14] He clearly separates the provision of medical care from a commodity transaction and emphasizes the helping role of medicine. The end of medicine should be service. Freidson's concern is that, without public-policy provisions, the commitment of the profession to service cannot be assured.

Freidson's view requires that we strike the delicate balance between regulations that assure compassionate service and the overregulation that stifles it. But without a moral commitment to beneficence by the physician, there is no certainty that even the best-calculated regulatory system will not be sabotaged. The trust built into the really critical decision in medicine can be assured only by the trustworthiness of the physician's character. This is an irreducible fact. The redirection of the physician's commitment that Freidson hopes for depends on a reformation of the physician's ethical sensitivities: regulation is a coarse adjustment of commitment; ethical sensitivity is the finer adjustment.

VOCATION AND CAREER

The internal morality of medicine can be distorted when the profession is regarded as a career, and perfected when it is regarded as a vocation. If it is a career, there is little justification for the higher degrees of beneficence we have emphasized throughout this book. On the other hand, if it is a vocation, even the high orders of beneficence might be insufficient. A career implies the cultivation of an occupation for personal ends and purposes—for power, prestige, personal satisfaction, influence, money, or immortality. These may be subsidiary ends in a true profession, but never the primary end. Self-interest, however "enlightened," will eventually conflict with the patient's interest at some point. In pursuit of a career, only so much altruism as will enable one to get ahead is permissible.

It is a career orientation that leads some physicians to refuse to treat AIDS patients, the poor, the alcoholic, or the rejected members of our society. This, they say, is not in their "contract" with society. They assert their right to treat or refuse to treat whomever they wish. For them, medical knowledge is proprietary—a personal possession to be used for personal profit, prestige, or power. They worked hard to acquire it. It is theirs to dispense. Society and the sick, they argue, have no overriding moral claim on them. Besides, society is now treating the doctor badly and the profession has a right to retaliate.

This viewpoint is directly counter to the idea of a profession as defined here. The latter is several steps higher on the ladder of ethical sensitivity. In its highest form it is tantamount to a secular vocation—a calling to a way of life dedicated to service of others.

For the Christian, a vocation presses for an even higher level of moral sensitivity. In its most general sense, a vocation is the call by God to all persons to seek salvation. Some accept that call; others may not. But all are called and receive the gift of grace that makes a response possible. In a more restricted sense, a vocation is a call by God to spend one's life in a particular set of circumstances, of which an occupation is one component. The call is to transmute any occupation, however humble or mundane, into an act of grace and charity to serve God in whatever one does as a means to personal salvation and service to others. For some this calling may be derived from other religions. For still others, the calling itself may have a non-deistic base. A religious conviction is not a necessary condition for a professional calling. We are simply illustrating what a profession is by looking at the possible religious basis of one's call.

For the Christian a profession becomes a vehicle through which beneficence is raised to the level of agape—an intent to live the message of the Sermon on the Mount. A Christian vocation recognizes the obligation to beneficence implicit in the internal morality of the professions. But it strives to elevate it to conform to the unselfish love manifest in the life of Christ. A vocation, while recognizing the limitations of human nature, is nonetheless a call to strive for perfection in charity in whatever one does.

The philosophical notion of profession therefore stands halfway between the higher obligations of a vocation and the lower obligations of a career. This distinction becomes a little clearer when we examine how one or two of the current moral challenges would accord with these three conceptions of the professional life.

Let us take first the example of care for the poor, the social deviant, and the handicapped and elderly. For the physician who sees medicine as a career only, there is no obligation to provide service for someone who cannot pay, who does not comply fully with the physician's orders, who is ill kempt and distresses the other patients in the waiting room, who continues to drink, smoke, or overeat, who is of a different social class. Such people drain resources, time, and energy to which they are not entitled. They deserve little because they are the chief sources of their own ill health. One might, out of condescension, help some of these people, but one has no obligation to do so. So goes the response of a troubling number of physicians (lawyers, and, sadly, some ministers) for whom their profession is an occupation, a career or a business.

On the other hand, if being a physician is truly a profession in the sense defined here, the moral response to this class of patients is different. One does feel a moral obligation, within limits, to assist those who cannot pay, to help at least some of them through free care in the office, clinic, or hospital, and to be an advocate on their behalf with policy makers, legislators, and society in general.[15] This degree of solicitude is built into the internal morality of the professions. It is to the credit of the traditional professions that the best among them have always exhibited this kind of solicitude.

If medicine, in addition, is seen as a Christian vocation, then one is bound to go several steps beyond. To follow medicine as a Christian vocation is to make a preferential option for the sick, the poor, and the dejected, to extend the notion of beneficence to the point of effacement of self-interest, indeed to recognize the "hard" message of the Gospel, the message that some unselfish sacrifice, as in the parable of the Good Samaritan, is required.[16] Obviously not all Christians are called to the level of sacrifice of a St. Francis, a Mother Teresa, or a Father Damien. But lesser degrees of charity are morally required. No one can prescribe for another what that degree should be. What is clear is that in a Christian vocation, something more than the internal morality of medicine is required. Exigencies and self-interest do not exonerate lapses in charity. Practice of the profession is an occasion for witness to what it means to be a Christian. A Christian vocation converts a profession and a career into an evangelical and salvific instrument.

At this point we must emphasize that many non-Christians and nonbelievers provide better examples of beneficence and solicitude than professed Christians. For them medicine is a secular "vocation." They are also in some sense graced. They show that the higher levels of beneficence are possible on naturalistic grounds, and they challenge Christians to show what further solicitude, compassion, and care are incumbent on those who profess to be Christians.[17] The question of a distinctive "Christian ethics" is, for many theologians, a debatable matter.[18]

THE MORAL DRIFT AND MORAL PHILOSOPHY

Given the ambiguous state of professional morality today, what may we expect for the future? Will the downward shift in moral sensitivity toward a career rather than a professional orientation continue? Can the descent be halted? Should it be? By what means?

To begin with, we must acknowledge that there has never been a golden era in which physicians were all committed to the high ideals implicit in the internal morality of medicine. Only a small number of physicians, for example, were committed to the Hippocratic ethic in Greek times. The majority were more attuned to a craftsman-businessman ethic than to a true professional ethic. Even fewer have practiced the profession of a Christian vocation.

For the future welfare of patients and the public, two matters are of grave importance: the number of physicians who opt for each of the three modes of professional life, and the degree of moral legitimation given to the career model and the self-serving ethic it fosters. If the majority of physicians were to choose a career model and if it were to gain moral sanction, then the character of medicine would change materially to the disadvantage and even peril of patients.

Beneficence and fidelity to the patient's interest would no longer be the moral standard. Without these moral underpinnings the rules of the marketplace and the pluralistic ethics of law and business would predominate. This puts patients, in the vulnerable state of illness, at the mercy of the least common ethical denominator. It would erode both the social contract that permits discretionary use of freedom by the professional and the moral imperatives that hold the normal human tendency toward self-interest in check. All of society would suffer diminution if the professions, which are among society's few examples of altruism, were to disappear.

The conflict between self-interest and altruism, between the professional and the career models, is bound to continue. The hope for the future is that the ethical sensitivities of professionals can be raised so that a larger number opt for a professional over a career mode. Professed Christians already have a mandate to conform to the vocation model.

The rule of the marketplace is profit, market dominance, efficiency, productivity, and monopoly. The customer is induced to buy, the weaknesses of one's competitor are exploited, and the entrepreneur is exalted. No one expects the merchant, banker, or salesman to think of the good of the customer or of effacing self-interest. The internal morality of the marketplace is simply inconsistent with just those notions that are intrinsic to the idea of a helping profession.

To legitimate the marketplace or career ethic is to deny the moral claims of patients on physicians, claims that arise out of the four characteristics that give the physician-patient relationship an obligatory moral quality.

Another danger lies in the public backlash to the abuses already beginning to appear in the marketplace ethos, e.g., economic transfers, rationing by ability to pay, revival of proprietary hospitals, and the reemergence of multiple levels of quality, accessibility, and availability of service. Calls for more stringent regulatory legislation are already surfacing. While some regulation is essential to patient welfare, too much is damaging. A vicious cycle soon ensues—abuses spawn regulation, and regulation limits the discretionary latitude of both physician and patients and bureaucratizes the experience of illness.

The conflict between altruism and self-interest is not a new one. The physician has always been torn between the good of the patient and his or her own family's need for financial security, recreation, and relaxation. It cannot be eradicated from any one of the three models we have been discussing. But if it is to be constrained by moral purpose, then self-interest cannot be given moral legitimation as a primary motivation for a life in medicine, nor can perfection of one's technique or the acquisition of knowledge. The moral legitimation for the clinician must always be the welfare of the patient. This is why there must be a moral shift back to the concept of a profession and, for the Christian, of a vocation.

How might this shift be accomplished? Manifestly, what is required is the moral awakening of as many physicians (and other professionals) as possible to the internal morality of their professional lives. We speak of an awakening, not a reawakening. We have no reason to suppose that medical students, physicians, and lawyers of today are in any way generically less moral than their predecessors. The moral shift lies in the legitimation of alternative models of professional morality. Any reversal in the direction of this shift must begin with a critical assessment of its conceptual foundations.

This calls for a genuine moral philosophy for medicine. This is distinct from the resurgence of medical ethics, which is well under way. Medical ethics—or biomedical ethics—in practice, if not in theory, is largely an exercise in conceptual analysis, as we have pointed out, in dilemma- and puzzle-solving and in casuistry in its best sense. This is necessary to the practical resolution of the many ethical conflicts in medical and professional ethics today. But medical ethics presupposes a larger framework, a moral philosophy that encompasses what we mean by morality, why we take certain positions, how we should live and why.

A moral philosophy for the professional would, at a minimum, set out a theory of medicine, of the professional, of healing, of the nature of the physician-patient relationship, and of how the physician should live life as a physician. A moral philosophy of law or ministry would do the same for these professionals. A starting point for all is a moral philosophy of the professions—something we have tentatively examined earlier in this chapter.

The seminal texts in medical ethics have not been treatises on moral philosophy. The most influential—such as the Hippocratic ethic—have been statements of morality without systematic or formal argumentation or justification. Even Percival's *Ethics*, which so deeply influenced Anglo-American ethics, is a statement of duties rather than a moral philosophy of medical duty. It is only in Percival's other writings that we can discern the moral philosophy that underlies his ethical precepts.

The current conceptual drift in the idea of professions underscores the need for a more explicit philosophy of the professions. Some ordering principles are necessary if we are to discriminate and decide which among the competing notions of a profession should be normative and why. This is a necessary first step. But given the philosophical pluralism of the times, the possibility of a universally accepted moral philosophy is not likely. Still, there are several advantages to an attempt to give it more explicit form.

For one thing, the underlying structures of competing ethical viewpoints will be more fully exposed. When there are conflicts, this should help to locate where they arise, which are negotiable, and which are grounded in nonnegotiable principles or beliefs. An explicit and conscious moral philosophy would help professionals to understand the reasons for their moral choices and those of their patients. In this era of patient autonomy, such mutual understandings are essential to the morally defensible conduct of physician-patient relationships.

Moreover, many physicians today are accommodating to the career model out of exigency. Critical and closer examination of what such a choice implies might dissuade some or at least give them pause. Many, of course, might still opt for that model. But the conscious realization of why one chooses one way of professional life over another should diminish self-deception. A more open and honest declaration of how one conceives of the professional life should diminish the deception that now hovers over physician-patient relationships in for-profit medicine or managed health care systems.

Further, the move to more public discussion and involvement in professional morality requires more formal explanations of why certain moral decisions are made rather than others. Individual physicians, lawyers, and institutions can expect to be asked to declare their positions—and the philosophy underlying them. More educated patients, clients, and parishioners are demanding to know, in advance, what kind of person and what kind of professional they are confronting. More and more, the choices of a professional institution are being made on the basis of its moral belief systems.

All of this is appropriate in a mature, democratic society that does not have a morally homogeneous value structure. It is also important to any profession that clings, even in the most tenuous way, to the appellation "learned." We no longer interpret "learned" to mean a physician literate and classically educated in the Oslerian mode. But we should retain the more fundamental idea of professionals as educated persons, i.e., those who are critically reflective about themselves, their way of life, their profession, and their moral choices. This is a minimal definition of education. Without it, the physician's identity is reduced to the techniques he or she employs—a choice some physicians may prefer. If they do, their pretensions to an education should be punctured.

The vocation model of a profession is also based in a moral philosophy that needs further explication. What is the meaning of a Christian vocation to medicine? What obligations does it entail in addition to the internal morality of a profession? How should the Christian live his or her professional life? What should the physician's response be to the drift to entrepreneurism, proletarianism, careerism, free-market principles, and the like? How compatible, if at all, are they with Christian moral philosophy? Is a Christian ethic possible?[19] We have provided some answers to these questions in this book, but we believe that they are only the beginning of a more explicit examination of the tasks of physicians in the twenty-first century.

Those same questions should apply to the idea of a profession as vocation in non-Christian systems. Judaism, Islam, Buddhism, and Confucianism—each has a moral philosophy that is linked to a way of life in medicine. The similarities and differences in these moral philosophies and their relationships with medical practice and moral choice are important to understand in our morally polyglot American society.[20]

For the good of patients and society, we may hope that more critical examination of the foundations of professional morality will slow the drift toward careerism and stimulate a reascent of moral aspirations. Whether this will occur or not is problematic. On balance, we expect that moral reexamination will, in fact, shift the vectors, in that those physicians whose instincts are to have a more elevated notion of professional obligation will get the reinforcement they seek and need.

Some physicians will, in good conscience, choose the career model nonetheless. If they make this explicitly known to colleagues and patients, their position will be more defensible than it is now, when the public expectation is still that they are adhering to the traditional model of a profession. While we might argue with the careerist's choice, we would have to respect the honesty of it. At least the patient will be alerted to pay heed to the ancient warning—caveat emptor.

A more explicit moral philosophy would make it clear to those who feel impelled to practice medicine as a vocation that many of the things legitimated today—the emphases on cost containment, entrepreneurism, the free-market philosophy, and libertarian notions of justice—are simply not morally defensible. For the Christian, it would be hard to reconcile Nozick's notion of justice with the Sermon on the Mount.[21] Nozick's conception of justice would deny that "the losers" in the natural lottery have any moral claim on the rest of society. For the Christian, this is precisely the group—the poor, the sick, the retarded—for whom a preferential option is required. Many practices now legal—especially those that derive from the concept of medicine as a business or industry—are mainly marginal at best. Yet they are defended even by many Christian physicians—a separation of professional and spiritual life inconsistent with the most rudimentary notion of a Christian vocation.

At this writing there seems little possibility that all the commitments formally included in the physician's ethical codes of the past will be restored. The moral diversity of our times makes that impossible and even undesirable. Clearly, some of the precepts of the past need changing; others should be nuanced, and others restored.

But even with the breadth of moral beliefs characteristic of our day, the development of an acceptable philosophy of the professions seems possible. For those who see medicine as a vocation, such a philosophy provides a starting point from which they must move to the higher requirements of agape. For those who see medicine as a career, it should provide a restraining force to those crasser motives that defeat the healing enterprise.

The moral and conceptual drift in medicine is occurring in law, ministry, teaching, engineering, science, and many other activities that see themselves as professions. Each in its own way faces the same challenge—to resist the downward moral drift that makes the use of specialized knowledge a danger instead of a boon to human welfare.

NOTES

1. Albert Camus, *The Plague*, trans. Stuart Gilbert (New York: Alfred A. Knopf, 1948).

2. These are a few examples. They have become symbols of the moral failure of professions. They are obviously not all of the same degree of gravity, but they indicate a progressive deterioration in the moral behavior of those upon whom so many depend and whom they are forced by circumstance to trust.

3. The deontological books of the Hippocratic corpus are The Oath, On the Physician, Precepts, On Decorum, and Law. See Ludwig Edelstein, *Ancient Medicine: Selected Papers of Ludwig Edelstein*, ed. Owsei Temkin and C. Lilian Temkin (Baltimore: Johns Hopkins University Press, 1967), pp. 328–329.

4. See Edmund D. Pellegrino, "Foreword," in Thomas Percival, *Medical Ethics, or a Code of Institutions and Precepts Adapted to the Professional Conduct of Physicians and Surgeons* (Birmingham, Ala.: Classics of Medicine Library, 1985), pp. 1–65.

5. "The Hippocratic Oath," in *Ancient Medicine*, ed. Temkin and Temkin, p. 6.

6. This is a phrase used by Harvey Cushing in an address in 1926. See Harvey Cushing, *Consecratio Medici and Other Papers* (Boston: Little Brown, 1929), pp. 3–13.

7. Robert Jay Lifton, *The Nazi Doctors* (New York: Basic Books, 1986). This is a devastating study of the rationalizations of physicians who played essential roles in German death camps. It is unequivocal evidence not of a moral drift but of a moral landslide.

8. These are just a few of the cases that have been the subject of litigation and widespread publicity in the last decade.

9. Ernest Greenwood, "Attributes of a Profession," *Social Work* 2, no. 3 (1957): 45–55.

10. Talcott Parsons, *The Social System* (Glencoe, Ill.: Free Press, 1951). Also "Professions," in *International Encyclopedia of the Social Sciences*, ed. David L. Sills (New York: Macmillan, 1968), pp. 536ff.

11. Martin S. Pernick, "Ethical Professionalism," in *Encyclopedia of Bioethics*, vol. 3, ed. Warren T. Reich (New York: Macmillan/Free Press, 1978), p. 1029.

12. Edmund D. Pellegrino, "Toward a Reconstruction of Medical Morality: The Primacy of the Act of Profession and the Fact of Illness," *Journal of Medicine and Philosophy* 4, no. 1 (1979): 32–56.

13. Ivan Illich, *Medical Nemesis* (New York: Pantheon, 1975); Jeffrey L. Berlant, *Profession and Monopoly: A Study of Medicine in the United States and Great Britain* (Berkeley: University of California Press, 1975).

14. Elliot Freidson, *Doctoring Together: A Study of Professional Social Control* (New York: Elsevier, 1975).

15. Erich Loewy, *Ethical Dilemmas in Modern Medicine* (Lewiston, NY: Edwin Mellon Press, 1988), pp. 33–56.

16. Laurence O'Connell, "The Preferential Option for the Poor," in *Medical Ethics: A Guide for Health Professionals*, ed. John F. Monagle and David C. Thomasma (Frederick, Md.: Aspen, 1988), pp. 308–317.

17. Edmund D. Pellegrino, "Health Care: A Vocation to Justice and Love," in *The Professions in Ethical Context: Vocations to Justice and Love*, ed. Francis A. Eigo (Philadelphia: University of Villanova Press, 1986), pp. 97–126.

18. Edmund D. Pellegrino, "Percival's Medical Ethics: The Moral Philosophy of an Eighteenth Century English Gentleman," *Archives of Internal Medicine* 146 (November 1986): 2265–2269.

19. Dennis J. B. Hawkins, *Christian Ethics* (New York: Hawthorn Books, 1963); Charles E. Curran and Richard A. McCormick, eds., *The Distinctiveness of Christian Ethics: Readings in Moral Theology*, vol. 2 (New York: Paulist Press, 1980).

20. For one example, see J. David Bleich, "The Obligation to Heal in the Judaic Tradition: A Comparative Analysis," in *Jewish Bioethics*, ed. Fred Rosner and J. David Bleich (New York: Sanhedrin Press, 1979), pp. 1–44.

21. Robert Nozick, *Anarchy, State, and Utopia* (New York: Basic Books, 1974).

7

A Community of Healing

This chapter examines the care and concern people should have for each other in human communities. Besides the natural basis of healing through a community of healers, we will also examine how and why religiously sponsored institutions are considered healing communities within the larger human community and why they must survive without moral compromise. Philosophy alone cannot provide the justification needed by such institutions in the present climate of cost containment, cost-effectiveness, competition, and a parsimonious social policy.

The task of healing, while it has its immediate focus in the individual sick person, nonetheless entails a community of healers, as we already suggested in chapter 4. If the members of that community are in conflict with one another, or the community is otherwise flawed, the healing task becomes difficult or even impossible.

Religious communities of healers build upon the natural community. It behooves us to briefly describe what we mean by the healing community before proceeding much further. The natural healing community is that group of people chosen by the patient on the basis of either professional or natural skills to provide the care and cure (if possible). Recall that we agreed with the notion that caring is a way of being in the world effected principally by assuring the patient about the stress of illness. Articulating that stress and helping to choose options to overcome it is a basic mode of caring for the sick person. Another way of putting this is that sick persons must turn to others officially or unofficially designated as healers. These persons, acting in concert with others, effectuate healing by addressing, through their own personhood, the suffering the patient experiences.

The ancient adage "Physician, heal thyself!" contains the seeds of this insight. Healers reach out into others' lives to help them reconstitute their values and their life plans during and after a disease or accident. This role cannot be totally fulfilled by technological means. Cures can be brought about this way, but the assault on the person requires personal involvement from the healer and his or her art. The healer must know something of suffering, what it is like to be confined to a wheelchair, what it is like to lack the funds for a taxi for the next scheduled visit, and what it is like to experience intractable pain.

What we have described thus far is the natural community of healers, one bound together by nonreligious values. A religious healing community is held together by commitment to specific values. This may take the form of a religious hospital or home health service. For Christian communities or, analogously, for other religious viewpoints, fidelity to a religious commitment defines the community over and above the natural instincts of healing. This lends such an institution a special healing character. Sometimes this character is almost palpably present. At other times it appears only as a faint afterthought.

Today spiritual healing communities confront serious economic, moral, social, and political conflicts inimical to their religious character. Indeed, unless these communities, as instantiated in health care institutions, adapt or compromise with secular value systems, they are threatened with fiscal failure or rejection by the larger communities in which they practice. In the interests of survival, they may compromise or even abandon their religious character. When they do so, they may enter Faustian compacts that inevitably must be paid off. The payoff spells disaster for their special mission in health care.

As a result, some hospitals have closed. Others have decided that it is not profitable to care for the poor or for complicated and expensive cases. Others are willing to provide only technical, short-term care. When the money runs out, patients are "dumped," an unfortunately blunt term for pushing patients out to those few public hospitals still operating, or to religiously sponsored institutions that are still trying desperately to fulfill a spiritual mission. Failing this, the patient too often is sent home to a family ill equipped to cope with the illness or the individual. Continuity, personalization, and individualization of care is fast disappearing as either a goal or an actuality.

Many hospitals today suffer from increasing entrepreneurial pressure. Some distressed hospitals, desperate for patients, are "offering bribes to ambulance drivers for each [Medicaid or insured] patient they bring in."[1] Entrepreneurship in health care is now an ethical problem, since physicians may own part or all of the laboratory or clinic to which they refer their own patients,[2] although laws have been passed that limit their ability to refer patients to their own clinics or businesses and still receive compensation.[3] These are two examples of the kind of internal destruction of the mission of healing that can take place in our society. From the strictly secular and economic point of view, entrepreneurship is just a smart business practice. But from the point of view of the healing task, it would be antithetical to any morally defensible ordering of values.

Yet what can a religious health care system do when caught in the squeeze between commitment and economic realities? When Medicaid funding in the State of Illinois ran out April 27, 1988, hospitals that cared for the poor faced a severe crisis.[4] Some closed. One of them was St. Anne's, on the west side of Chicago in a very poor neighborhood. Almost 70 percent of its care was provided through Medicaid and Medicare. The commitment of this Ancilla Systems hospital, in the face of the state's cutoff, could no longer be sustained. As the president and CEO of Ancilla Systems said in "An Open Letter to the Community": "It is no longer accurate to predict that we are headed for a crisis in the area of health care and delivery of hospital services, for we have already reached the crisis point."[5] Significant in this regard is that when religious communities of healers cannot accomplish their special mission, it becomes a problem for the whole community.

Changing social conditions create new identity crises and corresponding new opportunities.[6] Among the new opportunities are two major ones. First is the preferential option for the poor. One could well imagine that religious health care might become a "benefit" for those who practice their faith by becoming active in a parish or in the hospital itself. In this schema, health care would go first to those who helped in this ministry or in the larger church. This would fit into the institution's original conception of serving a specific population, e.g., immigrants, Catholics, Lutherans, etc. One could also imagine a church making a conscious decision to engage in the health care ministry and *not* seek the first place for its members. Rather, the first would be last, and the last first. The poor and the outcast would receive first access to health care.

There are real dangers in this approach, however. The main one appears to be that health care might be used as a coercion to join a particular church. "If you are converted and baptized, we will give you an injection to cure your illness." It would be morally repugnant to "sell" religion like cornflakes in this way. The second opportunity has to do with ownership. Some hospitals were sold by the religious communities that owned them. But is a ministry such as health care a thing to be sold, or a work of mercy over which one only has custodianship? The answer to this question is clouded by the fact that so many members of orders and congregations are retiring that the sale of the hospitals they own is the only way to support the care of their elderly religious.

These are only a few of the problems encountered by religiously sponsored health care institutions. A deeper question remains. Can the community consider healing others as optional?

IS HEALING AN OPTION?

In a profound way, the origin of all sickness is social.[7] Disrupted relationships, environmental decay, poverty, and pollution are all equal partners in causing and conditioning illness. Sin, social disruption, and sickness, as we saw in chapter 4, can be close allies in generating a context for illness.

It should be indisputable that the health care ministry will always be a primary apostolate for Christians. Sources for this assertion are plentiful in the Old and New Testaments, in the lives of Christ and the saints, and in the history of the Church. Moreover, hospitals as we know them today were, like the university, born in the bosom of the medieval Church and under the Church's aegis spread throughout Europe, and later North and South America and Africa. Many hospitals in America were founded by European religious orders, by churches, or by Jewish congregations. They were founded in remote regions or poverty areas, bringing medical care to otherwise unserved populations. In many communities these hospitals are still the primary source of medical care.

The contributions of religious hospitals to the health of America are yet to be appreciated by social and medical historians. For example, today 10 percent of hospitals and 15 percent of beds are under Catholic auspices in this country, with total expenditures of $15.5 billion.[8] Like other religiously sponsored institutions, very few of these hospitals are free of fiscal worries. For many, survival is so central a concern that it becomes a principle of decision making. Some of these hospitals, as a result, have been transferred to the community or sold to multihospital systems or for-profit corporations. The challenge these institutions face is to maintain an authentic religious health care ministry while avoiding the distortion of that ministry by the fiscal exigencies of today's socioeconomic and moral climate. Some of the fiscal maneuvers devised by hospitals faced with declining occupancy clash directly with a mission to care for the poor. They pose a serious threat to the religious character of the healing mission and contravene the very idea and meaning of a healing community.

Concerns for the proper care of the elderly and other more vulnerable members of society raise questions about their moral claims on the common resources of society. If those resources are scarce, how may one justify their preferential application to the most vulnerable, rather than equitably to all? Can this source of claims on the goodwill of others be derived from philosophical or political principles, or does it in fact reflect historical values derived from a religious viewpoint about society and the goals of human life?

It is one thing, as Hume pointed out, to acknowledge the natural state of affairs about scarce resources. It is quite another to ask what resources society plans to make available in pursuit of its aims of justice.[9] If everyone received everything they ever imagined they needed, there would be little point in debating issues in social justice. But in reality, this discussion appears in every society because of what Hume called "limited benevolence."[10] The limits we place on social resources for just causes betray our fundamental convictions about the dignity and value of individual persons in society.[11]

What therefore is the ultimate justification for the claim that the sick have a moral right to health care? Is it just that we should be linked to others? Why is it that healing only comes about through human relationships? Cures of diseases might be possible through medical technology alone, but the healing of persons depends on bonding with other human beings. These are crucial questions for a moral philosophy of health care, and they are yet to be answered definitively.

THE CHALLENGES

Forty years ago, religious hospitals seemed a permanent fixture on the American scene. Their major responsibilities then were to improve the quality of their services and make them consistent with a religious vision of the healing ministry. They were confident of their place in a healing and helping ministry that extended back at least to the Middle Ages in the case of Catholic health care. Doubts regarding identity, authenticity, and continuation were not entertained. Yet a mere forty years later these are precisely the questions that are the most pressing. Does fiscal survival demand too many compromises with the essential spirit of a religious ministry?

Of the many changes over the past forty years, three in particular stand out for their effect of eroding the spiritual character of the health care ministry. They are a decline in vocations (in Catholic health care), commercialization and competition, and the general moral pluralism of our culture.

Decline in Vocations

Religious communities of sisters and brothers were the backbone of most of the Catholic health care ministry. The progressive decline in vocations to the religious life means that the centuries-long presence of sisters and brothers at the bedside of the sick is lost. Today that presence is diminishing to the vanishing point. The few remaining religious are increasingly pulled into administrative and managerial roles. They are forced to become, sometimes willingly, entrepreneurs, skilled at wrestling with the competition, lighting more votive lights to Adam Smith than to St. Jude. Often that competition comes from another religious hospital in the immediate area as it vies for patients with a sister institution. Both attempt to deny the other the limited number of patients available.

Because of their dwindling numbers, many religious institutes have been forced to sell their hospitals as their major capital asset. The money from these sales is needed to build endowments for their aged, ill, and retired members. Some traditionally health-oriented congregations have asked whether health care and the healing ministry represent the best use of their depleted personnel. More talented members have been placed in high-paying jobs outside the health ministry to sustain the community's finances. As a consequence, many religious hospitals are under lay management and are staffed by individuals who are not committed in any particular way to the religious vision of the founders.

Nothing is intrinsically wrong with these trends. It is important to become more efficient in the delivery of health care. Some hospitals will have to close. But these trends demand a deliberate restructuring of what is essential to the healing task in order to maintain a specifically religious character. One conclusion is inescapable. All members of the hospital must share a vision of healing, beyond mere curing, that can maintain the special character of the institution. This represents a golden opportunity to involve more people in an ecumenical, nonsectarian examination and implementation of "caring for the whole person." Formerly individuals who shared this vision were content to let it be represented by religious leaders, sisters, brothers, chaplains, rabbis, and the like. Now the vision must be "enstructured," to coin a word. It must become part of the very protocols of healing the sick.

Commercialization of Health Care

Even if there were a sudden and dramatic reversal of this trend and religious and volunteer health workers became abundant, the integrity of a religious mission of healing would be threatened by the recent sharp change in American attitudes about health care delivery. About twenty-five years ago, health care came to be regarded as a right of all citizens (though it was never proclaimed as such). At that time the rhetoric of policy makers and politicians was filled with promises of equity in quality, availability, and accessibility. National health insurance was always "just around the corner."

Though none of these ideals was ever achieved, the nation did gradually begin to close the gap in health and medical services among its citizens with the advent of social programs for the poor and elderly. With Medicare and Medicaid, programs for mothers and children, and a variety of other special federal programs, the two-level system of medical care was on the way to elimination. So much was this the case that most city and county hospitals for the medically indigent either closed entirely or reduced their beds drastically.

As the cost of these programs escalated in the seventies, rhetoric became more restrained. Now it was "quality care at a cost we can afford." Alternative modes of delivery, such as HMOs and outpatient medical and surgical care, were promoted to keep patients out of hospitals. Hospital lengths of stay decreased, and the days in the hospital became more costly as all forms of tertiary care were expanded.

With the beginning of the eighties, concern for costs came to dominate the thinking about health and medical care. Equity and rights no longer appear very high in the discussions. Instead health and medical care are seen as commodities like any other, to be purchased in a competitive market. Medical knowledge is the property of providers, to be sold to those who can pay for it. Price, availability, and quality are to be determined by competition among providers, whose self-interest (it is presumed) will bring cost and quality into favorable balance.

As a result of the failure of competition to bring down costs (health care continues to expand faster than the general rate of inflation), health care expenditures are now an inviting target for budget balancing. Corporations eye their contributions to health benefits while increasing the employee share. The government is openly circumscribing Medicare and Medicaid benefits. The elderly are taxed unfairly for the burden of catastrophic care. The poor and the medically indigent, we are told, must learn to accept minimal levels of care and forgo the higher technologies available to those who can pay. The same is true of the elderly. The return of the municipal and county hospital two- or three-tiered system is almost inevitable in light of these budget battles, thus returning us to a system of health care we had worked hard to eliminate in the last forty years.

In the past, hospitals used to charge those who could pay, or their third parties, more than it cost for their care in order to underwrite care for the indigent. This "Robin Hood" system has now vanished as the wealthy, third parties, and corporations imitate the government in squeezing escalating health care costs to the minimum. Hospitals can no longer charge the well-to-do to care for the poor. Charity care must be funded in some other way. Religious hospitals feel this problem as secular ones do, but the funding for the care of the poor cannot be demanded of society unless such hospitals behave like secular institutions (or at least are placed at risk of losing their identity).

Health care has become, in the apt words of Eli Ginzberg, "monetarized."[12] For-profit hospitals and health care corporations are gaining an ever larger part of the "market." Health care is a "growth industry" and an "investment opportunity," rather than an essential service and an obligation to citizens to be provided by a civilized society. Capital expenditures must come from bond issues, and bonds are rated, of course, on the bottom line. Even the idea of a profession, a group in society dedicated to something other than self-interest, is subordinated to the primacy of competition.[13]

Religious hospitals, in consequence, are forced to compete on terms inimical to their mission of preferential treatment for the poor and disadvantaged.[14] They find themselves drawn into "survival tactics" like establishing for-profit subsidiaries, forming networks with institutions whose moral principles differ from their own, or proffering treatment on the ability to pay rather than on need for care. These practices are justified by the fact that without a profit margin, there can be no mission at all since the alternative is fiscal failure and extinction.

Is there any realistic way to allocate care in response to religious, rather than secular, motives? If the resources of society for health care are truly limited (in our judgment, a proposition not yet proven), is there a way to preserve the idea of a healing and caring community? Must the religiously sponsored hospital accept, accommodate, and adjust to the "realities" of a competitive marketplace in health care? Or, is there an obligation to act singly and in cooperative arrangement with other religiously inspired institutions, not only to resist these realities but to create alternative systems more consistent with Christian ideals of healing and helping the sick? Competition is useful for many commodities that are best distributed by the marketplace. But health care is not a commodity. The task of healing, and particularly of Christian healing, is not reducible to a commercial transaction.

Moral Pluralism and Participatory Democracy

The third challenge strikes at the heart of a community of healing. Essential to the healing mission is the creation of a hospital that is itself a healing community—an "operative Christian community" in the sense that John Paul II used that term to apply to Catholic universities.[15] Broadening it to cover all religious hospitals would mean that the commitments of the original charter and the commitments that are explicitly and formally designed into the mission and philosophy statement are operative, that is, put into practice. As such, a hospital would require all its members to put into action a unified dedication not only to providing quality health care in the spirit of charity but also to helping each member of the institution grow spiritually. It must exhibit charity in its relationships with staff and the community it serves, as well as with the patients and their families. If it be operative, it must be open to God and the guidance of prayer even in its economic decisions. Indeed, the stories of the founding of these hospitals invariably contain elements of crisis and economic desperation.

Management and sound fiscal responsibility are always moral imperatives in a religious community. Religious hospitals must exercise these qualities, too. But unlike a secular institution, they must be modulated by solicitude for the poor, the outcast, the aged, the seriously ill—for all those who live in the shadows of modern life and are the easy victims of an unrestrained competitive, entrepreneurial spirit.

A religious healing community is also one that clearly and unapologetically provides care within the framework and tradition of religious moral principles. The importance of these principles in today's ferment in medical morals is obvious. The religious teachings should guide the operation of the healing community in regard to social justice, abortion, sterilization, euthanasia, newer reproductive technologies, and the care of the dying, the incompetent, or the congenitally defective infant. What the institution does with respect to these issues may vary considerably from those of contemporary society.

Can such religious institutions be faithful to specific ethics in their healing ministry in the face of moral pluralism in a democratic society? Can a religious hospital truly be a "community" hospital, if the people it serves do not share its religious commitments? What if its moral values diverge too much from the constituent population? Many who staff a religious hospital do not share the moral teaching of the sponsoring religious organization. Often the method by which a plurality of views is protected is procedural rather than substantive. This is part of the American genius. The "melting pot" theory of American culture holds that many different moral points of view and many divergent cultures have been joined together in one basic culture. But this is not the case. Americans enjoy a free concourse of ideas, but they have not been "melted" together, to say the least. The way usually chosen out of moral conflicts is to develop procedural rather than substantive ethics. This advances the peaceful settlement of morally opposed positions. A good example is the report of the committee formed to recommend to the director of NIH whether or not aborted fetal tissue could be used in research. The "consensus" was overwhelmingly in favor of its use. But such a procedural process cannot erase the underlying substantive ethical issues, i.e., possibly encouraging and benefiting from elective abortions, objectifying a form of human life, placing utility ahead of other moral principles, and demeaning the moral status of the fetus itself in the human community. We explore this issue further in chapter 9.

THE JUSTIFICATIONS

Justifying continued existence as a religious community providing healing beyond care is an important new process. As we already noted, what was once largely provided realistically and symbolically through sisters, brothers, and other religious leaders must now be structurally designed into the institutions themselves. All members of the institution must discuss these commitments and carry them out as far as possible (in light of their own conscience as well).[16]

The Dignity of Human Life

There can be no serious question of a retreat from the health care mission. Indeed, the very factors that threaten this mission constitute the moral imperative for its continuance. Religious health care institutions are the only reliable safety net when government policies and national attitudes, both often quite fickle, turn away from the poor, the medically indigent, and the losers in the competitive milieu we value so highly. To espouse a religious commitment without offering material help under these circumstances is duplicity of a particularly unsavory kind.

Today's exigencies are created less by a scarcity of resources than by a disinclination to share them. We are moving toward a two-class society in which Dives and Lazarus no longer even see each other. Being religious means making a difference in everything that is done. Simple acquiescence to the world as it is is not a sufficient answer to the evangelical obligations "people of the Word of God" all share. As Pope John Paul said: "The parable of the Samaritan of the Gospel has become one of the essential elements of moral culture and universally human civilization. . . . No institution can by itself replace the human heart, human compassion, or human initiative."[17]

Human Life as Social

To be human is to be intimately social, in the deepest part of our being. And to be social is, in part, to be linked not only to all other human beings through hope and despair, through aspirations and disappointments, through life and eventually death, but also to be dependent on those other humans in our life. No one likes to be reminded of her own dependency, but this is the ineradicable message of all serious illness. Our selves and our bodies are put in the hands of others. We are, quite literally, forced to rely upon other persons with the presumed expertise to help us.

Essential, but difficult to develop and assess, is the conscious promotion and practice of the spirit of charity and concern that give to religious hospitals their special solicitude. That solicitude is manifest when the hospital grows into a genuine healing community. Then there is mutual recognition that certain commitments to persons on a more profound level than is normally the case between "providers" and "clients" exemplify the care a community offers to a dis-eased person and family. This, too, is a lesson in community.

Institutional Integrity

Equally demanding is the necessity to provide institutions in our culture that reflect and support the fundamental beliefs of specific communities in society. Nothing can be more disruptive of healing than to be forced, while one is sick, to defend one's deeply held values—religious, philosophical, and cultural. Instead the sick person needs the help of professionals and institutions that will reinforce the values of the one who is sick. In such institutions, persons can be assured that their beliefs will be respected and they will be protected from pressures to conform to secular values. In those sensitive and stressful moments when crucial life decisions are being made, patients, their families, and those who serve them will need the spiritual and moral support a healing community can provide. Caring physicians, nurses, and other health workers, such as social workers and chaplains, are found in secular institutions, too. But by the nature of these institutions reaffirmation of religious or spiritual values is fortuitous at best and not a moral mandate by charter and public commitment.

The Most Vulnerable

This analysis can begin by citing the principle of vulnerability. By it one is required to give more to those who need more, to balance the imbalanced relationship occurring when one becomes ill and seeks help from others who are relatively healthy. In a previous work on the philosophy of medicine, we derived an axiom regarding vulnerability from the nature of medicine itself. We argued that, in order to attain the goal of medicine, healing, several ethical axioms were required, the violation of any one of them being inimical to the goal.[18] Respect for vulnerability was one of these axioms. Patients are at a twofold disadvantage in relation to the healer. First, the patient needs the physician in order to become healed (even if the work of healing is done by the patient). Second, the patient is in a position of unequal power. These two impediments to full self-determination are inescapable phenomena of the predicament of illness.

The healing community responds in a special way to the predicament of vulnerability. To those who suffer, it gives more of its material and emotional resources. We can think of the costs in dollars, human effort, and emotional support society expends rescuing a trapped miner, effecting a liver transplant for an infant with biliary atresia,[19] or comforting the victims of natural disasters.

Of these and similar responses we can as humans be justifiably proud. Such actions reflect a "deeper humanism," one that Pope Paul VI defined as a humanism that is "complete and seeks the full development of the whole personality of every man."[20] This humanism is a transcendent humanism. For religious persons, human beings are not the final definition of themselves. There is more to human life. Paul VI said: "Far from being the ultimate measure of all things, man can only preserve himself by reaching beyond himself."[21] In his first encyclical, *Redemptor Hominis*, Pope John Paul II gave voice to similar sentiments in his explication of the meanings of Christian humanism.[22]

SECULAR AND "SACRED" HEALING

There are similarities between a secular healing response and a religious one. It serves little purpose to attempt to show that a religious perspective has "trickled down" into secular ethics so that such responses become second nature to us. Rather the difference seems to lie in the realm of obligation. A secular society is not obligated to maximize efforts on behalf of the most vulnerable. Some conceptions of justice may even make such efforts appear to violate the rights of others. This is the libertarian argument of Nozick and Engelhardt.[23]

But a religious community of healing cannot take this position. In such a community each individual is endowed by his or her Creator with an intrinsic dignity and worth that demands respect. A true healing community under the fatherhood of God calls forth an expanded view of our obligations to other individuals. This intensification of our natural instincts and training is precisely what St. Thomas encompassed in his conception of the supernatural virtues.[24] His view was that grace built upon nature, it did not destroy it. This intensification of the strength of our obligations on behalf of others is what characterizes a religious perspective on healing.

A religiously inspired principle of healing might be stated this way: the greater the vulnerability of a human being, the greater protection we ought to afford. "The first shall be last, and the last first." This is a derivation from the religious expansion of the principle of justice. In this view, the impediments to equality of respect, in an ideal community, ought to be removed by the members of that community. Civil rights, for example, are a sign of a healing community, not just a set of negotiated entitlements. A healing community must care for those it succors.

The care of the disabled is a case in point. Socially responsive care of the disabled presupposes a kind of society in which the most vulnerable are protected by the more powerful. Outside such a society appropriate policies that support those in greater need cannot be established. The powerful would protect themselves at the expense of the most vulnerable. In many respects, we have cause to reflect on our frightening closeness to a Nazi society whose attitudes toward the disabled, handicapped, or racially outcast were uncomfortably suggestive of some of our own.

HEALING AS PROPHETIC

Our focus on the prophetic aspects of healing is grounded in the New Testament, although they are rooted in Old Testament traditions. The healing acts of Jesus were not just significant for the individual. Much has been made of the structure of the stories of healing in the New Testament. The desperately sick individual obtains relief by an appropriate act of faith, a renunciation of past sinfulness, and a response to a future hope.

But in the context of the New Testament message, healing and the announcement of the presence of the reign of God go hand in hand. Jesus commands his disciples to heal the sick and preach the Kingdom of God (Mk 6:7–13; Matt 10:1–15; Lk 9:1–6; 10:1–20). As Lambourne points out: "To heal the sick and to preach the Kingdom are neither complementary, nor supplementary, but both are manifestations of the same word of God. When Jesus confronts men and women with powerful acts of healing he does not ask for mere wonder and awe; what he asks for is that men and women will recognise in the healing act a theophany, God's presence, his word, his finger."[25]

Thus, healing is a prophetic activity, a proclamation of the presence of the reign of God in human affairs. Lambourne again says: "In the mission and message of Jesus Christ his healing work was not a secondary consequence, but the very means of the proclamation, institution, and enlargement of the new age, the rule of God."[26]

Healing is a community act for an individual or a populace that not only repairs disruptions at the individual and social level but points to the presence now of a distant and mysterious reality. This reality is the coming reign of God in human affairs, a perfectly healed community. In this eschatological vision, all disruptions are repaired. The body is transmogrified, not as a primary cause of the healing but as an effect of it. The resurrection itself is the ultimate sign of the presence of this new community of grace breaking into human history, the ultimate victory of life over death, hope over despair.

What is important about healing actions are that they are public signs. Not only are they significant for the individual; they are significant for the kind of response they evoke in the community. Are they a sign of God's presence? Do they draw persons closer to the eschatological vision? The reign of God comes upon the community within its midst.[27] Dodd called this "realised eschatology," meaning that the presence of the Kingdom was proclaimed in its immediacy. Later scholars modified this notion to "imminent eschatology," stressing instead the public-sign nature of the healing act, how it points to the future as well.

The community is in the sick person just as the sick person is in the community.[28] The sick person represents the community. Foulkes puts it this way: the sick person presents in his or her disease "the interacting network of human relationships from which it grows."[29] To present oneself to be healed is to ask the community to heal itself. The community of healers is at once the community of healing. This is a quasi-sacramental reality.

THE COMMUNITY OF HEALERS

If the process of healing effectuates and demonstrates a new kind of age in the history of human beings, an age in which the human person thrives in freedom and love because the community thrives in freedom and love, then the eschatological reality of the healing process signifies for Christians a different kind of community of healers than that envisioned by libertarians and other philosophers.

The usual focus of philosophic concerns about individuals in the health care system is on the relation of the vulnerable person to increasingly powerful interventions. Arguments are advanced to empower individuals within this alienating environment to maintain a measure of control over their own life and destiny. Health professionals are encouraged to promote patient autonomy as an essential step in the healing process, one in which the individual regains command of his or her own life.[30] This point of view is valid and important.

In addition, however, the Christian vision of the healing process introduces concerns about the healing community itself. First and foremost, the healing community must bring about healing rather than just cure. This leads to a different set of concerns from those traditionally addressed by philosophy, concerns about what happens to healing professionals who encounter the power given them by technology. A Christian cannot choose not to share his self with others through the healing process. Both physician and patient must share the human frailty and the suffering of knowing we have to die, in order that liberation of the person occurs in healing.

Thus the profession of medicine, among others, is a profession called to establish community by either eliminating or overcoming the barrier to community that illness represents. To do this, we must transcend the merely biological possibilities.

DUTIES OF THE COMMUNITY OF HEALERS

The call to establish community of service can reach all persons, even if it does not have specific sectarian content. This is very important in developing unity of purpose in a religious health care institution while recognizing the religious and secular pluralism of the staff. Just as Jesus' Sermon on the Mount functions for Christians as an ethics beyond philosophical ethics, so too must a religious community of healers articulate a set of duties that transcend the biological caring duties common to all human beings, common to the natural healing community. As Richard McCormick puts it for Christians:

> The Christian story tells us the ultimate meaning of ourselves and the world. In doing so, it tells us the kind of people we ought to be, the goods we ought to pursue, the dangers we ought to avoid, the kind of world we ought to seek. It provides the backdrop or framework that ought to shape our individual decisions. When decision making is separated from this framework, it loses its perspective. It becomes a merely rationalistic and sterile ethic subject to the distortions of self-interested perspectives and cultural fads, a kind of contracted etiquette with no relation to the ultimate meaning of persons.[31]

Examples of specific Christian duties might include the following:

1) The vulnerability of individuals must be respected. Beyond treating everyone equally, with equal respect and equal access to care within the institution, greater attention will be given to those with greater needs.

2) The capacity to suffer pain distinguishes all animals from lower levels of life. Animals have the necessary biological sensorium to experience pain. It is debatable whether lower animals can actually "suffer." While all higher animals experience pain, suffering is the physical, emotional, and rational response to both the meaninglessness and meaning of pain. Loewy argues that animals also suffer because they demonstrate appropriate stimuli and responses to events such as their master's death.[32] We think this view may be influenced by too much anthropomorphism. Be that as it may, the capacity to heal this suffering distinguishes human beings from other animals. This capacity can be seen through the eyes of faith as humanity's share in the very essence of God's power to rejuvenate and restore creation. Hence, a religious principle of healing requires transcending biological and technical means of care.

3) The preferential option for the poor is not simply an "option" for Christians. It is an obligation to choose to care for the poor to a greater extent than that found in secular society.[33]

4) The rule against killing is firmly embedded in the Christian tradition. This means that active euthanasia and abortion ought never to be permitted. Assisted suicide, as a form of active euthanasia, is also

ruled out. In place of killing, a Christian healing community ought to focus on compassion and responsiveness to the pain and suffering of individuals in its care.

A Christian and a secular humanist may come to the same conclusions about these duties of one human being toward another. They are desirable goals for the whole community. Arguably, these duties and others can be deduced from human nature itself. But for the Christian, these duties are required by charity. They are not optional or honorific. The Christian cannot use utility as an excuse not to treat individuals, for example, even though Mill argued that utilitarianism was the most Christian of ethics. This has bearing on hospital practice with respect to institutional survival and the care of the poor.

Of the levels of professional and personal duties toward one another, there are at least four, three of which are circumscribed by a Christian perspective.

The Biological Level: Health care professionals have a fundamental and role-specific duty to aid persons suffering from distortions of biological function due to disease or accident. The goal of duty at this level is reversal of disease or accident and restoration of function. The challenge is to deal with the person as a holistic organism, not just a conglomeration of body parts and systems. That is to say, the person should be treated as a subjective as well as objective entity.

The Covenantal Level: Health professionals have an additional duty, not necessarily role-specific, that derives from the contract, implied or explicit, with the patient. In part the contract requires health professional commitments to the good of the patient, now not narrowly conceived as a biological good alone but as a kind of life-good.[34] With respect to the role-specific duty the contract obligates professionals to compassion and altruism. There is a social contract within this level as well, stemming from the expectations of society regarding training and support of health professional education, experimentation, licensing, and so on.

The Existential Level: Health professionals have a requirement to deal with the patient in all his or her relations, including the relation to life itself. Here the goal of care is not just to treat the whole organism that is a person, but the person's values and relationships with respect to life, others, the family, work, and society and culture itself. The best way to articulate the goal of care at this level is to say that health professionals have the obligation of trying to achieve for each individual the basis for the purposefulness of life, that is to say, sufficient health to pursue other, more important, values. The goal of medicine, therefore, is not prolonging life at all costs but, rather, honoring life as a conditional good.

The Theological Level: Essentially the theological level of duty is that of one creature toward another, in humble acknowledgment of the mystery of life. Here the goal of care is not so much to achieve an end produced outside life and the relationship between the doctor and the patient as it is to achieve an understanding of joint human frailty, of the vulnerability of being a creature destined to die. Put simply, the goal here is compassion, suffering-with. Each patient is a brother or sister.[35]

CONCLUSION

The religious basis of health care can contribute insights into general theories of medicine that do not require that persons accept a particular faith or belief system. As we saw, the natural duties inspired by faith are defensible in general terms as a good for the whole community. Healing communities can articulate these duties by attending to the nature of human suffering and our common capacity to heal.

Yet for religiously inspired healing communities, these duties are not optional. They are required by their moral vision. The calling of these communities to follow a religious vision of the human community helps them derive their obligations to the sick from a transcendent ethic of compassion, justice, and charity. Further, society in general, and religious communities in particular, expect more of communities of healing than they do of other institutions.

At root, the religious healing community should pay particular attention to the more vulnerable, in whom through their affliction "God is working."

NOTES

1. Katherine Eban Finkelstein, "Bellevue's Emergency," *New York Times* (February 11, 1996), Sec. 6, p. 45.

2. Michael Weinstein, "The Clash of Ethics, Law, and Economics over the Issue of Patient Referrals," *American College of Physicians Observer* 9, no. 4 (1989): 1, 10–11, 13.

3. David C. Thomasma, "The Ethics of Medical Entrepreneurship," in *Health Care Ethics: Critical Issues,* ed. John F. Monagle and David C. Thomasma (Frederick, Md.: Aspen, 1994), pp. 342–350.

4. "Medicaid Funding Cut Off by State," *Chicago Tribune* (April 27, 1988): 2, 3.

5. Alethea O. Caldwell, "The Health Care Crisis: Its Impact on the Communities We Serve," *An Open Letter to the Community* 1 (periodic publication of Ancilla Systems, 1100 Elmhurst Rd., Elk Grove Village, Ill. 60007).

6. Laurence O'Connell, "The Preferential Option for the Poor," in *Medical Ethics: A Guide for Health Professionals,* ed. John F. Monagle and David C. Thomasma (Frederick, Md.: Aspen, 1988), pp. 271–280.

7. Robert A. Lambourne, *Community, Church, and Healing* (London: Darton, Longman & Todd, 1963), pp. 1–10.

8. Catholic Health Association of the United States, *Facts about the Catholic Health Association of the United States [Fact Sheet]* (St. Louis: Catholic Health Association, 1996).

9. David Hume, *An Enquiry Concerning the Principles of Morals* (Indianapolis: Hackett, 1983).

10. Hume, *Enquiry.*

11. Robert E. Goodin, *Protecting the Vulnerable* (Chicago: University of Chicago Press, 1985), pp. 1–15.

12. Eli Ginzberg, "The Monetarization of Medical Care," *NEJM* 310, no. 18 (1984): 1162–1165.

13. Edmund D. Pellegrino, "What Is a Profession? The Ethical Implications of the FTC Order and Some Supreme Court Decisions," *Survey of Ophthalmology* 29, no. 3 (1984): 1–15.

14. O'Connell, "Preferential Option," pp. 306–312.

15. Pope John Paul II, "Address" (Washington, D.C., Catholic University of America, Oct. 7, 1979).

16. Kevin O'Rourke, O.P., J.D., has outlined clearly the justification, role, and responsibilities of lay cooperation. He goes so far as to characterize the laity's apostolate in the Catholic Church as the "hope" that will ensure continuance of the Church's presence in health care. See Kevin O'Rourke, *Reasons for Hope: Laity in Catholic Health Care Facilities* (St. Louis: Catholic Health Association, 1983).

17. Pope John Paul II, *Salvifici Doloris* (Washington, D.C.: United States Catholic Conference, 1984), pp. 36–37.

18. Edmund D. Pellegrino and David C. Thomasma, *A Philosophical Basis of Medical Practice* (New York: Oxford University Press, 1987), ch. 7, pp. 155–69.

19. See Jack Houston, "Nine-Month-Old Meghann LaRoccco, Youngest Person to Receive Four Liver Transplants," *Chicago Tribune* (March 14, 1987), sec. 1, p. 5.

20. Pope Paul VI, *Populorum Progressio* (Washington, D.C.: United States Catholic Conference, 1967), p. 36.

21. Pope Paul VI, *Populorum Progressio.*

22. Pope John Paul II, *Redemptor Hominis* (Washington, D.C.: United States Catholic Conference, 1979).

23. Robert Nozick, *Anarchy, State, and Utopia* (New York: Basic Books, 1974); H. Tristram Engelhardt, Jr., *The Foundations of Bioethics* (New York: Oxford University Press, 1987).

24. St. Thomas Aquinas, *Summa Theologiae,* vol. 23, trans. W. D. Hughes (New York: McGraw-Hill/Blackfriars, 1969), I–II, art. 62, responses 1–4, pp. 137–145.

25. Lambourne, *Community, Church, and Healing,* p. 42.

26. Lambourne, *Community, Church, and Healing,* p. 35.

27. Charles H. Dodd, *The Parables of the Kingdom* (London: Hodder & Stoughton, 1936).

28. Lambourne, *Community, Church, and Healing,* p. 43.

29. Siegmund H. Foulkes and E. James Anthony, *Group Psychotherapy* (New York/London: Penguin Books, 1957), p. 78.

30. Eric Cassell, "Autonomy and Ethics in Action," *NEJM* 297, no. 6 (1977): 333–334.

31. Richard A. McCormick, *Health and Medicine in the Catholic Tradition,* vol. 3 (New York: Crossroad, 1987); Martin E. Marty and Kenneth L. Vaux, eds., *Health/ Medicine and the Faith Traditions: An Inquiry into Religion and Medicine* (Philadelphia: Fortress Press, 1982), p. 50.

32. Erich Loewy, *Suffering and the Beneficent Community* (Albany: State University of New York Press, 1990).

33. O'Connell, "Preferential Option," pp. 312–317.

34. Edmund D. Pellegrino and David C. Thomasma, *For the Patient's Good: The Restoration of Beneficence in Health Care* (New York: Oxford University Press, 1988).

35. Edmund D. Pellegrino, "Every Sick Person Is My Brother and Sister," *Dolentium Hominum, Year III* 7 (1988): 65.

8

Love and Justice in the Health Ministry: From Profession to Vocation—Philosophical Perspectives

Perfect charity is perfect justice.

St. Augustine, *De natura et gratia*, LXX, 64.

In this penultimate chapter and in the final chapter, we will try to coalesce the ideas presented so far, with special attention to the specific obligations that the Christian health care ministry must adopt if it is to remain true to its calling. Adopting these obligations moves health care from a profession to a true vocation.

INTRODUCTION

The Questions

Love and justice are two virtues without which peaceable and civilized societies cannot exist. For non-Christian societies, they are dictates of reason; for Christian societies, they are dictates of reason illuminated by faith. The spiritual challenge to all Christians is to live these virtues as they have been transvalued by the gospel message.

Nowhere is the test of love and justice more urgently met than in the care of those at the margins of society—the very young, the aged, the poor, the oppressed, and the depressed. We may declare faith in the Christian message, but unless love and justice eventuate in charitable justice, an authentic Christian life is not possible. As Augustine puts it, "For without charity, faith can be, but profit nothing."[1]

We wish to examine the ways in which Christian perspectives on love and justice should shape our attitudes and behavior to the sick— ways in which scriptural, ecclesial, and episcopal teaching supplement and complement individual and societal obligations deducible by reason alone. What differences do Christian conceptions of love and justice make in the ethics of the health professions? What transforms a health profession into a Christian vocation to the health care ministry?

The scope of such an enquiry is unmanageable in any definitive way. It is essential, therefore, to practice at least some economy to limit the subject. For one thing, we shall not derive or cite the extensive biblical or scriptural sources for Christian conceptions of love and justice.[2] Nor shall we review the content of episcopal and ecclesial documents, for reasons we underscored in our introduction.[3] Finally, we will also skirt the exquisitely important question of the distinctiveness of Christian ethics. The differences, some sharp and some subtle, among the Church's most distinguished theologians on this point are sufficient to inhibit all but the most temerous commentator.[4] Nor are these debates the point of this book. Suffice it to recall directly Jeremiah's exhortation to do justice to the vulnerable (Jer 22:3), Sirach's warning not to avert our eyes from the poor (Sir 4:1–5), Jesus' dedication to his mission to the poor, the blind, the captives (Lk 4:16–19), or the obligations of Christians to go beyond mere justice (Lk 6:32–35).

We will delimit this chapter in still another way, and that is to concentrate on what is currently the most urgent confrontation with the principles of love and justice for Christians and non-Christians— the challenge of economics and the marketplace to the altruistic spirit that both faith and reason dictate in the care of the sick. We have decried the intrustion of the marketplace into the values of health care throughout the book and will not concentrate on the religious rationale behind that judgment.

The Problem

Christian churches and Christian communities have never been so directly challenged as they are today by fiscal expediency to compromise the Christian call to love and justice. For the last two decades, and especially in the last five years, the tendency has been to translate a legitimate concern for the rising costs of health care into a justification to commercialize and monetarize the care of the sick. The thesis is advanced that subjecting health care to market forces—competition, advertising, consumer choice—will control costs and demand and assure quality as well.

An outcome of the market mentality is to reduce health care to a commodity transaction, making it a service to be purchased like any other. Distribution, access, and availability of health care are left to the rules and ethics of the marketplace. The ancient medical ethical principles of beneficence and justice are thus to be reinterpreted in terms of economic utility.

In this view, medical ethics tends to be equated with the minimalist ethics of law and business transactions. The effacement of self-interest and the altruism traditionally expected of health professionals are eroded as profit-making and entrepreneurship are legitimated. The tension between altruism and self-interest is not new to the medical profession. What is new is the encouragement of professional self-interest as a respectable motive with social utility.

Christian health professionals, physicians, nurses, dentists, and administrators cannot help being touched in fundamental ways by these forces. They are already embracing the metaphors of a commodity transaction—an industry instead of a ministry, entrepreneurship instead of vocation, and adequacy instead of equity. In the interests of fiscal survival many are accommodating to, or compromising with, the monetary mores of contemporary health care. The crucial questions are: How far may they go without losing their religious identity? How consistent is the industrial and commodity model of health care with the Christian concepts of love and justice?

Are the only alternatives survival at the expense of moral compromise or moral authenticity at the expense of extinction? Can religious denominations responsibly avoid the dilemma by retreating from the health care ministry as some have already done and others are contemplating? Much depends on the essentiality of care of the sick to the Church's evangelical mission. Is health care, or is it not, a necessary call to all Christians to witness the difference the good news of the gospel makes in human affairs?

The Method

The content of these questions is, in part, philosophical and, in part, theological. The answers are central to any formulation of contemporary medical and bio-ethics. It is fortunate, for this effort, that these fields are enjoying an unprecedented flowering just at this time. The thrust of this flowering is philosophical, and this is proper for the morally pluralist, democratic society in which we live. The Christian, too, must begin his examination philosophically—by the use of reason, unaided by revelation.

As we have taken pains to point out, for the Christian, philosophical bioethics is not enough. For one thing, the dominant spirit of contemporary ethics is analytic rather than normative.[5] It eschews ultimate normative principles except, perhaps, utility or freedom. It is, as a consequence, difficult, if not impossible, to validate morality itself or to select among competing ethical theories and ethical norms. Christian theological ethics, however, does provide ordering principles derived from revelation, and it links ethics with the sources of meaning of human existence. It is a necessary supplement to philosophical ethics if a complete medical morality is to be found.[6]

For these reasons, we must ascertain the ethical content of health and medical care philosophically first, and this calls for an enquiry into the two central principles of philosophical medical ethics—beneficence and justice—together with the obligations that flow from them. Then it is necessary to inquire into the transformations of the meanings of benevolence and justice, their shaping by the fact of revelation. Finally, one can then examine the central question by using the Christian concept of charity-based justice as a principle of discernment in confronting some of the concrete issues in medical-care ethics today. With these as principles of discernment, the moral commitment of Christians to love and charity is translated into concrete acts, decisions, and choices in personal and social ethics. A profession becomes a vocation to the health ministry when its actions are in conformity with Christian ideals of love and justice.

We shall argue on both philosophical and theological grounds that the concepts of love and justice are inconsistent with the ethics of the marketplace, that all society is diminished when health care becomes a commodity and altruism is subverted by self-interest. In addition, we shall argue that Christian understandings of love and justice go beyond the naturalistic interpretations and provide principles of discernment that shape the responsibilities of health care ministry for individual professionals, the institutional care of the sick, the formulation of health policy, and the relationships of the institutional Church and the people of God to health and health care.

We hope to emphasize perceptions that might be common to the whole Christian community. Our argument, it is hoped, will not lose its force for those who differ on these fundamental points.

The argument applies to all health professions, not just medicine. For simplicity's sake, however, we shall use the term "medicine" broadly to stand for all the healing professions—nurses, dentists, allied health workers, as well as physicians—a practice we have employed throughout this book. This is not to argue that the term "physician" subsumes the others or that they do not have independent standing; by concentrating on the physician's role, however, we can make the enquiry more specific.

The chapter is divided into two sections. They are argued philosophically under two subheadings: I) "The Nature of Illness and Healing" and II) "The Root Principles of Philosophical Medical Ethics. In our final chapter, the last three parts of our argument are presented theologically under three subheadings: I) "The Theological Perspective," II) "Christocentric Health Care Ethics: From Profession to Vocation," and III) "The Call of the Whole Church to the Healing Ministry."

THE NATURE OF ILLNESS AND HEALING

Then, isn't it the case that the doctor, insofar as he is a doctor, considers or commands not the doctor's advantage but that of the sick man?

Plato, *Republic*, I, 342, D.

We begin with what is deducible from reason about beneficence and justice so that we can more clearly discern what is added by the Christian counterparts of these two principles. Justice and beneficence are, after all, ancient virtues cogently and extensively expounded in pre-Christian times and exemplified in the loftier aspirations of ancient and classical medical codes. They are not discoveries limited to Christianity but have been, and are, open to all who possess human reason. Indeed, the practice of beneficence and justice by pre-Christians or non-Christians has, far too often, exceeded in sincerity and genuineness that manifested by some Christians. Still, when interpreted authentically,

Christian conceptions of justice and beneficence in medical care are different in inspiration and content from even their higher manifestations in non-Christian sources.

Since our inquiry into love and justice is focused on their expression in health care, we must look at the central phenomena of illness and healing, which give health care its moral qualities. Here we review our reflections from the early chapters of the book. The first question is whether illness is a special kind of human experience. If we are to argue against the increasingly prominent view that health care should be treated like any other commodity or service, then it is necessary to show wherein being ill differs from other human experiences—at least in degree, if not in kind. This requires some operational definitions of health, illness, and healing—three concepts under vigorous discussion among philosophers of medicine.[7] These concepts can be fully defined only if we have a coherent theory of medicine.[8] Such a theory is not yet fully developed. We have attempted an introduction to such a theory elsewhere.[9] Some features of that effort are called up in the discussion that follows.

Let us start with the empirical and phenomenological aspects of illness. In this view, "illness" is the subjective perception of a person that he has experienced a change from the customary state he regards as health. "Health" in this context refers to a patient's own interpretation of that state of functioning that permits him to do the things he wishes to do with a minimum of pain, disability, or restriction.[10] The person's perception of a change in existential states from health to illness is crucial, whether the change is acute or perceived over a period of time. The state a person regards as health need not be one free of disease or demonstrable disability. One may feel well and function even in the presence of manifest or covert pathological processes. Contrariwise, one may feel ill in the absence of a demonstrable structural or functional abnormality.

"Health" here refers therefore not to some ideal state of freedom from all social, physical, or emotional dysfunction. Rather, it is a state of balance, an equilibrium established between inborn or acquired diseases or limitations and the use of our bodies for transbodily purposes—to advance personal interests, plans, or aspirations. Each of us strikes such a balance, which for us defines our personal definition of "health." The idea of health as balance is more analogous to the classical notions of *eukrasia*, *isonomia*, or *sōphrosunē* than it is to some quantitative calibration of objective health determinants and measurements.[11]

Taking this subjective view of health and illness does not militate against assessing more objective criteria and remedying or preventing deviations from statistically defined criteria of normality. Nor does it preclude cultivating higher or better states of balance by positive health promotion. Rather, concern here is for a person's experiential perception of whether he is in need of healing—of a restoration to some previous state of affairs to which he had adapted and adjusted his life. At that precise point, when the person who feels ill decides that he needs professional help, he becomes a patient—one who seeks to be healed by another person who "professes" to heal.

The patient, as we already noted from the etymology of the word, "bears" a burden—a pain, a symptom, or a disability. These burdens he recognizes as threatening to his personal conception of health. Their presence shatters his sense of wholeness. He can no longer cope without assistance. Now, as a patient, the ill person presents himself to a health professional for advice, for relief of anxiety, for assistance in being healed, in becoming whole again, in returning at least to his prior state, if not a superior one.[12]

Illness signals a change in existential states in the most crucial ways since illness assaults the whole person. Even a trivial or easily remediable illness or injury carries with it some compromise in the operations of one's humanity. The ill person lacks knowledge about what is wrong, whether it is serious, whether it can be cured, how it will be cured, and at what expense in time, money, pain, discomfort, and loss of dignity and privacy. The ill person is also dependent on another for this information. She also lacks the skill and knowledge by herself to answer these questions and to effect the needed cure.

The ill person moreover has lost the free use of her body for her own transbodily purposes. Indeed, the body has in a sense revolted. It has taken the center of the stage. It demands attention. It demands to be served, rather than serve. The body stands against the self, it becomes alien. The ontological unity that constitutes the well-functioning human person is compromised or even ruptured. Illness thus threatens our image of self—the identity we have fashioned as a result of the balances we have struck between our endowments, great or small, and our aspirations. The image and the meaning we have given to our lives must often be reconstructed if healing is to occur. How will the illness change us? What new demands will it place upon us? Will it mean that, at last, we must confront the fragility of personal existence and the reality of personal death?

These phenomenological characteristics of the experience of illness converge to make the patient a changed person. He has become a dependent, vulnerable, and exploitable human being. The sick person remains, ontologically, a human being, of course, but the freedom with which he can express his humanity is limited. Illness is, as we said, a wounding of the humanity of the one who is ill. The sick person has lost some of those precious freedoms we associate with being human.

Healing requires nothing less than repairing these wounds. It calls for a restoration to the former or a better state. If this is not possible, healing strives for whatever balance is still possible. Even the patient who is incurably ill can be healed to some extent. She can be helped to grasp control of her own living, to the extent possible, to direct her own life, even in the face of obvious decline. She can be helped to regain some hope that her own death can be confronted in a human and personalized way. With assistance, the sick and dying person can refashion a new self-image, one that confronts dying or incurability in her own way.

These summary phenomenological observations give only a superficial statement of the changes in existential states that constitute illness, health, and healing. They should suffice to remind that being ill and in need of healing is a special state of human existence and that the particularities of the experience are unique for each human person. Since the story, the narrative of each life, is unique, the "continuation" of that story in the face of illness is also unique.

Let us now develop our case further. As a consequence of these reflections, illness is different in degree, and even to some extent in kind, from being in need of some material commodity or service. Illness strikes much closer to what it is to be human. Hunger, poverty, and injustice are states of deprivation, too. They share some of the phenomenological characteristics of illness. Yet they are, in a real sense, external assaults visited upon us by circumstances or other persons: They do not represent primarily internal and intrinsic attacks on a person's capacity for survival or for enjoying a satisfying life. Injustice and poverty limit possibility, but they do not eliminate them as illness can.

Health, or well-being, is an intrinsic human value. It is both a biological good—the well-functioning of the whole organism—and a social good essential to the well-functioning of society.[13] It is a different thing to be in need of healing than it is to be in need of some commodity—a refrigerator, a new car, or even a new job. Illness, if not a unique state of deprivation, is one that seriously undermines our capacity to live a fully human life, in ways that strike close to what it is to be a human being.

In this special state of deprivation, the ill person seeks out the healer. The healer, in turn, offers herself—that is to say, "professes" that she can and will heal. It is in the nexus of this personal transaction between one seeking help and one offering help that the ethical obligations of the healer are grounded. To promise to heal elicits expectations in the patient: that the physician will have the necessary competence, and that she will put that competence at the service of the patient. The very nature of illness, what it does to persons, and the nature of the promise to heal: together they create a necessity for trust. The physician must be the patient's advocate to warrant that trust. She has the obligation to practice a certain self-effacement, suppressing her own self-interests in favor of those of the patient. The physician must not use the vulnerability and exploitability inherent in the sick state to advance her own power, prestige, or profit.[14] She must be compassionate because she cannot determine the good for *this patient* without feeling something of this patient's experience of illness, the patient's perception of his own good in *this* clinical situation, at *this* time in his life.

These expectations are heightened by the existential inequality of physician and patient. This is not an ontological inequality, for the patient remains fully a human person—entitled to the full measure of respect due all persons. But illness imposes an existential inequality, since the patient is less free, less knowledgeable, less powerful than when he was well. His humanity is less free to express itself. His control of his own destiny is compromised, and he is forced to trust in the character and virtue of the physician.

In a sense, the physician is also less free. She is bound, by the promise to heal, to this patient in a bond of trust. This bond limits the full expression of her own self-interest. Her promise to heal limits her freedom to pursue what might otherwise be legitimate goals—profit, prestige, or power. The physician's bond is forged by the promise to help, a bond of a type inconceivable in a business or commodity relationship.

In that circumstance of inequality, the physician is expected to make a decision for, and with, the patient and take an action that is technically correct and morally good.[15] The two need not be, and increasingly are not, synonymous. Medical good does not exhaust the meanings of the patient's good. We can think of an expanding number of situations today in which the assessment of the physician and the patient differ about whether a recommended treatment is worthwhile—blood for the Jehovah's Witness, abortion for the Catholic, discontinuance of life support measures for the Orthodox Jew, any kind of nonspiritual healing for certain fundamentalist religious sects. Doing good for the patient is a complex act that calls for a balancing of techno-medical good (what benefits medical knowledge may bring) and the other dimensions of patient good—his preferences, his good as a human being to make autonomous decisions, and his spiritual or ultimate good.[16]

It is the confluence of these special existential aspects of illness, of professing to heal, and of healing itself that grounds medical ethics and gives it a special character within the broader context of human ethical behavior. Even on purely philosophical grounds, and without recourse to theological argument, the healing relationship transcends the buyer-seller relationship. Accordingly, the ethical obligations of patient and physician are of a different order from the obligations of buyer-seller.

It is those naturalistically deducible differences and specificities that ground medical morality and have in all major cultures enjoined higher degrees of commitment upon physicians than expected in other members of society. We find those obligations spelled out in most of the ancient and modern modes of medical ethics in the Judaeo-Christian West, as well as in China and India.[17] These codifications vary in content and may, at some points, contradict one another. Yet they all call for primary deference to the patient's well-being, for competence, for avoiding injury to the patient, and for respecting the vulnerability of the sick person.

Some will object that despite these lofty aims the medical profession has, in its individual members, so often and so egregiously lapsed that the idea of self-effacement is a myth and a sham. There is no doubt that transgressions of the medical codes have, sadly, been all too frequent. But that does not vitiate their intrinsic validity or the impressive fact that as many physicians have, in fact, honored these codes as have violated them—a record not equalled in any other endeavor except the religious ministry.

It is important for the major emphasis of this chapter—the meaning of Christian love and justice in the health ministry—that Christians appreciate the high level of aspiration, if not perfect adherence, that pre-Christian, pagan, and non-Christian medical ethics have attained. Benevolence and, less explicitly, justice are two virtues that civilized societies expect of their physicians for reasons that arise out of the nature of what it is physicians profess to do for those who are ill.

The challenge for Christians is to define what makes a Christian ministry of health care distinctive. What does it add to the loftier expressions of secular or non-Christian humanisms?[18] To examine that question further, we need first to look, still from the philosophical point of view, at the meanings of beneficence and justice inherent in the pre-Christian and non-Christian codes and in today's philosophical medical ethics.

THE ROOT PRINCIPLES OF PHILOSOPHICAL MEDICAL ETHICS

We have outlined the philosophical grounding of medical ethics from which the major principles of traditional medical ethics can properly be deduced. Those principles are reducible to two: beneficence (doing the good of the patient) and justice (giving to each one his due). The other principles usually employed are subservient to those two. Thus autonomy—the obligation to enhance and to permit the patient's right of self-determination and choice—is a component of beneficence, since doing the patient's good includes respecting his specific good, as he defines it, as well as his generic good, as a rational being capable of exercising reason and making choices.[19] Promise keeping, confidentiality, and truth telling can also be subsumed under a broadened conception of justice and/or beneficence.

Before we examine the ways in which the Christian conceptions of love and justice reshape the naturalistic conceptions of beneficence and justice, we must examine in more depth the explicit meanings of these two cardinal principles in contemporary philosophic ethics.

The Principle of Beneficence

Benevolence and beneficence—intending and doing the patient's good, i.e., acting in his or her best interests—is a complex notion.[20] The good of the patient subsumes at least four separate notions. The *first* is medical good—what the scientific and technological knowledge of medicine can effect to cure, contain, ameliorate, or prevent illness or disease. It consists in the judicious application of current medical knowledge and techniques. Its benefits are measured in terms of some quantitative effect on the unfolding of the natural history of the disease. Medical good in a given clinical situation is determined by "medical indications"—a statement of those clinical characteristics that make the application of a given therapeutic modality worthwhile in certain classes of patients. Worthwhileness implies some possibility of good that materially outweighs the dangers and discomforts of a particular treatment.

In some models of beneficence, the whole good of the patient is equated with medical good and is the doctor's only proper concern. This is the doctrine of strong paternalism, which holds that only the physician can know what is good for the patient, that the patient can never comprehend fully the risks and benefits, and that medical good is the only good the patient should seek from the physician.[21] Medical ethics, in this view, is measured by the canons of medical competence solely.

The *second* sense of patient good is the good as expressed in her preferences, her expressions of what she considers in her own best interests. This form of a patient good will vary markedly from patient to patient. It incorporates many values, the kind of life the patient would like to live, the risks she wishes to take, and for what benefits. Each of us has a life plan and a set of values arranged in some order of preference, some set of things we wish to achieve and things to avoid. These values are based in culture, ethnicity, age, sex, occupation, family, and dozens of other facets of our individual lives.

When illness occurs and alternative treatments or outcomes are presented, each of us may weigh the possibilities differently. Each of us therefore has a somewhat different concept of our own best interests. No one else can presume to define those interests for us or the quality of life we may wish to lead. In clinical decisions, therefore, the medical good recommended by the physician must be placed within a matrix of personal preferences and shaped accordingly, or even rejected.

When the physician encourages and permits the patient to make his own decisions, without deception or manipulation she respects the principle of autonomy. This principle is fast becoming the prime principle of medical ethics in our democratic, pluralistic, and free society.[22]

Autonomy is the *third* sense of the patient's good. It is a generic good proper to all humans as humans, as beings worthy of respect. It is grounded in the human capability for reason, choice, and judgment and in the capacity to express those choices in speech. Autonomy exercised in making moral choices becomes moral agency—the autonomous choice of a person among moral values and his accountability for the choices made. This is a good so intrinsic to being human that to violate it is to violate the very humanity of the patient, even if he chooses to refuse effective treatment and risks death as a result.

Much has been written about the patient's moral right to autonomy in contemporary medical ethics. It is placed by some authors in direct opposition to beneficence.[23] Those authors generally equate beneficence only with medical good. Taken this way, beneficence may indeed come into conflict with autonomy. But if beneficence is looked at more broadly, it includes preservation of patient autonomy, because the patient's good is not limited to his medical good. Autonomy and beneficence in this view cannot be in conflict.

The *fourth* sense in which patient good may be understood is as ultimate good. This is the "good of last resort," in the sense that when everything else is considered, this good predominates over all. This good is often expressed in spiritual terms and related to the final destiny of persons. For the preservation of good of the soul or its spiritual advancement, humans may sacrifice all the preceding senses of good. They may even yield up their autonomy as religious do in the vow of obedience, sacrifice their lives or goods for others, or deny or endanger themselves to help others.

Even those who reject spiritual beliefs will have a good of last resort, a good for which they may sacrifice all other goods. It may be a humanistic love of mankind, of country, the "greatest good" for all, the advance of science, the pursuit of utility, pleasure, nirvana, etc. Whatever it may be, ultimate good is the final ordering principle that will not be sacrificed in a crisis and will ultimately ground and justify moral choice.

We have arranged these four senses of patient good in an order of increasing hierarchical value. When they are in conflict, as they can well be, medical good is the least—and ultimate good the highest—good of the human person. We discuss this in detail elsewhere.[24] Briefly looked at here, beneficence, even on strictly philosophical grounds, is a prime obligation of the physician. Beneficence means that he must respect each component of his patient's good. Because of the phenomenological features of the physician-patient relationship (emphasized in section I), the physician has a role-specific ethical obligation of trust and fidelity to act beneficently. This obligation goes beyond nonmaleficence, which is simply not to do harm and therefore the most minimal construal of beneficence.

The Principle of Justice

The second great principle of philosophical medical ethics is justice, which, like beneficence, is grounded in what it is to be human. Aristotle puts it well: "Justice is essentially human, *i.e.*, it suggests the mutual relations of men as men."[25] Justice is usually defined in some variation of the ancient dictum *suum cuique*. This notion of rendering to each according to his or her due is intrinsic to the multitudinous definitions of justice advanced from book 1 of Plato's *Republic* to the contemporary influential theories of Rawls and Nozick.[26] Each definition contains something of the *suum cuique* notion, but different shades of interpretation can yield radically different products when expressed in concrete human behavior. These differences become most apparent later when we examine justice in the allocation and rationing of resources.

Classically, justice has three dimensions, each of which is important in philosophical medical ethics—commutative, distributive, and social. Since each is modulated in a Christocentric ethic, each deserves some discussion first in philosophic terms.[27]

Commutative justice concerns the private relationships of persons. It is rooted in the essential equality and dignity of the persons making agreements or contracts with each other. It demands fidelity to promises and agreements, and a lack of coercion. In such agreements one may not take advantage of the other, since the contracting parties are both equally human.

In medical relationships commutative justice requires fidelity to the trust necessitated by the nature of medical acts. It requires the keeping of promises made by physicians to patients. It preserves the covenantal nature of the physician-patient relationship. On the empirical bases set forth in section I, justice requires that the physician be faithful to the obligations implicit in her promise to help the patient. It includes truth telling as well, since patients cannot make free and personal

choices without knowledge of the nature of the illness and its progno-
sis. Justice follows from the necessity of beneficence in medical relationships. It takes on a special character, however, because physician
and patient are not really equal existentially, though both are still
human.

The second sense of justice is distributive. It covers the responsibilities we owe each other as members of a society, or community, the
claim each person has to some share in public goods even if his direct
participation in the production of those goods may be remote. This
claim arises from our mutual interdependence as social animals, each
of whom can be fulfilled only in a communal life. In contemporary
society, those common goods would include, for example, security,
social services, a clean, safe environment, protection of natural
resources, health care, housing, nutrition, etc. These are goods whose
distribution is required if each member of a human community is to be
a participant in that community. These are goods none of us could own
or enjoy in isolation from our fellows. None of these can properly be
considered "propriety" even in a capitalist society.

Health care is among those goods governed by the principle of
distributive justice, since without health, it is difficult or impossible to
participate in society. In this sense, health is a precondition of a fully
human life.[28] Likewise, it is difficult to conceive of a "healthy" society
in which a significant number of its citizens are not healthy. How distributive justice is to be made operative in our society is today the subject of the most vigorous debate. Some of the most crucial questions in
that debate are unanswered: What is the strength of the individual's
claim? Is health a legal right, an obligation of society, or a luxury allow-
able only if sufficient affluence permits? By what criterion of justice
shall health care be distributed? Should it be equity, merit, age, achieve-
ment, need, social worth, productivity, or ability to pay? What level of
distribution is justified? Shall it be access and availability to all health
services, to none at all, or to some specified "fair" minimum?

John Rawls's impressive effort to elaborate a philosophical theory
of justice emphasizes both maximum liberty compatible with the freedom of all and the distribution of social inequities in such a way as to
be to everyone's benefit.[29] "Injustice, then, is simply inequities that are
not to the benefit of all."[30] In Rawls's view, we do not deserve our fate
in the natural lottery. The ideal social contract is one in which we are all
equal unless inequality favors the least advantaged or increases liberty.

Rawls justifies his position on the basis of the "original position," the assumption that his is the contract we would choose if we did not know where in the natural lottery we would fall. Health care, in this view, would be distributed so as to advantage the less advantaged. It would favor egalitarianism and the establishment of social minimums for distribution and allocation of resources.

Nozick, on the other hand, interprets justice as preserving each one's entitlements, the advantages or disadvantages we receive in the natural lottery—our genetic, social, economic, and political endowments.[31] Society, in this view, is not compelled in justice to remedy the quixotic distribution of goods that results from the natural lottery. If some are less healthy, less favored economically, or more powerful politically, this may or may not be unfair, but it is not unjust.[32] Nozick's view applied to health care favors liberty, as does Rawls's. But in the distribution of inequities, goods, and resources, Nozick's favors nonegalitarianism. Nozick does not preclude a society voluntarily redressing the imbalances of the natural lottery. But he would deny to the individual a moral claim, in distributive justice, to amelioration of the disparate entitlements resulting from his unfortunate position in the natural lottery. This conception of justice emphasizes individual differences and a pluralist conception of the principle that constitutes distributive justice.

The third sense of justice is social—the shared obligation of the members of a society to fashion and operate institutions and arrangements that will fulfill the obligations defined under distributive justice. This is justice in its sociopolitical expression. It calls for the creation of agencies, institutions, systems, and structures that will take account of the mutuality and interdependence that ground distributive justice. Social justice is a necessary condition of distributive justice, for without it the claims of individuals for participation in society's goods cannot be realized. In this view, it is a mutual obligation of all citizens to foster the formation of social organizations responsive to the claims of distributive and commutative justice.

As applied to health care, social justice is in an even more vexed state than distributive justice. What is the most appropriate form of government, and what degree of government regulation would best foster a just distribution of health care? What limits can be placed on individual freedom and entrepreneurship in the interests of optimizing social justice? What are the relative merits of a free-market economy as opposed to centralized or planned mechanisms for health care distribution? How consistent are for-profit hospitals, the corporate practice of medicine, the licensing of physicians, the accreditation of medical schools, with a just distribution of health care? Clearly, some of the most crucial sociopolitical and economic questions of health care today turn on the interpretation we make of social justice.

CONCLUSION

Obviously, we cannot, in this chapter, attempt to answer these questions in any definitive way. This is by no means an exhaustive delineation of the senses in which justice may be taken. Compensatory and retributive justice, for example, have not been mentioned. They are important in health care and will be touched upon in the next chapter. What we have sought to establish is only the range of possibilities inherent in the concept of justice as it applies specifically to health care. The theories of Rawls and Nozick offer opposing, and even on some points contradictory, ways to interpret justice.

What is pertinent to our discussion is the way a Christian perspective on justice and benefience would influence our choices among these and other construals of justice derived philosophically. For this, we must turn now to the theological perspectives on love and justice.

NOTES

1. St. Augustine of Hippo, *Augustine: The Trinity*, trans. Stephen McKenna (Washington, D.C.: Catholic University of America Press, 1963), bk. 15, ch. 18, no. 32, p. 496.

2. Only a few of the summarizations need be cited: John R. Donahue, "Biblical Perspectives on Justice," in *The Faith That Does Justice*, ed. John C. Haughey (New York: Paulist Press, 1977), pp. 68–112; Monika K. Hellwig, "Scriptural and Theological Bases for the Option for the Poor," in *Justice and Health Care*, ed. Margaret John Kelly (St. Louis: Catholic Health Association, 1984), pp. 1–12; Laurence O'Connell, "The Preferential Option for the Poor and Health Care in the U.S.," in *Medical Ethics: A Guide for Health Professionals*, ed. John F. Monagle and David C. Thomasma (Frederick, Md.: Aspen, 1988), pp. 312–317.

3. See the excellent summary by Joseph Gremillion, "Papal and Episcopal Teaching on Justice in Health Care," in *Justice and Health Care*, ed. Kelly, pp. 31–43; and George Reed, "Initiatives of the Catholic Bishops in Seeking Justice in Health Care," in *Justice and Health Care*, ed. Kelly, pp. 45–59.

4. See the excellent multiauthored volume edited by Charles E. Curran and Richard A. McCormick, *The Distinctiveness of Christian Ethics: Readings in Moral Theology*, vol. 2 (New York: Paulist Press, 1980). See also Josef Fuchs, *Christian Ethics in a Secular Arena* (Washington, D.C.: Georgetown University Press, 1984); Richard A. McCormick, "Does Religious Faith Add to Ethics' Perception?" in *Personal Values in Public Policy: Conversations on Government Decision-Making*, ed. John C. Haughey (New York: Paulist Press, 1979), pp. 155–173; Garth L. Hallett, *Christian Moral Reasoning: An Analytic Guide* (Notre Dame, Ind.: University of Notre Dame Press, 1983); Robert J. Daly, et al. *Christian Biblical Ethics* (New York: Paulist Press, 1984); Patricia B. Jung, "A Roman Catholic Perspective on the Distinctiveness of Christian Ethics," *Journal of Religious Ethics* 12 (Spring 1984): 123–141. Kenneth A. Vaux, *Birth Ethics* (New York: Crossroad, 1990), examines issues in population and reproduction from the point of view of a multifaceted Christian ethics, arguing that the issues themselves point to the need for a broader normative reasoning process that characterizes such ethics.

5. H. Tristram Engelhardt, Jr., "Bioethics in Pluralist Societies," *Perspectives in Biology and Medicine* 26 (1982): 64–78; Alasdair MacIntyre, *After Virtue* (Notre Dame, Ind.: University of Notre Dame Press, 1981); David C. Thomasma, "The Possibility of a Normative Ethics," *Journal of Medicine and Philosophy* 5, no. 3 (1980): 249–259.

6. Edmund D. Pellegrino, "Religion and the Sources of Medical Morality," *Convergence* 2, no. 2, (1982): 33–40.

7. See Arthur L. Caplan, H. Tristram Engelhardt, Jr., and James J. McCartney, eds., *Concepts of Health and Disease: Interdisciplinary Perspectives* (Reading, Mass.: Addison-Wesley, 1981); see also the entire issue of *Journal of Medicine and Philosophy* 1, no. 1 (1976).

8. Pellegrino and Thomasma, *A Philosophical Basis of Medical Practice* (New York: Oxford University Press, 1987).

9. Pellegrino and Thomasma, *For the Patient's Good: The Restoration of Beneficence in Health Care* (New York: Oxford University Press, 1988).

10. Here we have paraphrased Galen's oft-quoted definition of health as that state "in which we neither suffer pain nor are hindered in the functions of daily life" (*De sanitate tuenda*, I, 5). Despite many wordier attempts, this simple definition has not been much improved upon.

11. See Henry Sigerist, *A History of Medicine*, vol. 2 (New York: Oxford University Press, 1961), p. 299. Also Werner Jaeger, *Paideia*, vol. 2 (New York: Oxford University Press, 1944), ch. 1. Plato's notion of health as a balance centered on his multiform notion of *sōphrosunē* —the orderly arrangement of faculties of the soul. See *Timaeus*, 87E–88A. The idea of balance between body and soul and the idea of *sōphrosunē* run through *Gorgias*, *Charmides*, and *The Republic* as well. See Edith Hamilton and Huntington Cairns, eds., *Plato: The Collected Dialogues* (Princeton, N.J.: Princeton University Press, 1961).

12. Edmund D. Pellegrino, *Humanism and the Physician* (Knoxville: University of Tennessee Press, 1979), p. 225.

13. Leon R. Kass, *Towards a More Natural Science: Biology and Human Affairs* (New York: Free Press, 1985), pp. 170–174; Joseph Owens, "Aristotelian Ethics, Medicine, and the Changing Nature of Man in Philosophical Medical Ethics: Its Nature and

Significance," in *Philosophy and Medicine*, vol. 3, ed. Stuart F. Spicker and H. Tristram Engelhardt, Jr. (Dordrecht, Holland/Boston: D. Reidel, 1975), pp. 127–142.

14. Pellegrino and Thomasma, *A Philosophical Basis*, ch. 7, pp. 155–169.

15. Pellegrino and Thomasma, *A Philosophical Basis*.

16. Edmund D. Pellegrino, "Moral Choice, the Good of the Patient, and the Patient's Good," in *Ethics and Critical Care Medicine*, ed. Loretta Kopelman and John Moskop (Dordrecht, Holland/Boston: D. Reidel, 1985), pp. 117–138.

17. For example, see the following: Hippocrates, "The Hippocratic Oath and Corpus," in *Hippocrates*, vol. 1, trans. W. H. S. Jones (Cambridge: Harvard University Press/Loeb Classical Library, 1972); H. A. Menon and H. F. Haberman, "From the Caraka Samhita," *Medical History* 14 (1970): 295–296; T'ao Lee, trans., "Five Commandments and Ten Requirements," *Bulletin of the History of Medicine* 13 (1943): 271–272.; Ariel Ba-Sela and Hebbel E. Hoff, "Isaac Israeli's Fifty Admonitions of the Physician," in *Legacies in Ethics and Medicine*, ed. Chester Burns (New York: Science History Publications, 1977), pp. 145–157. For an overview, see Burns, *Legacies in Ethics*; and Robert M. Veatch, "Medical Codes and Oaths," in *Encyclopedia of Bioethics*, vol. 3, 2nd ed. (New York: Macmillan, 1995), pp. 1419–1435.

18. For an example of some lofty Stoic sentiments, see Scribonius Largus's introduction to *Compositiones*, cited in Henry Sigerist, *Ancient Medicine: Selected Papers of Henry Sigerist*, ed. Owsei Temkin and Lillian Temkin (Baltimore: Johns Hopkins University Press, 1967), pp. 336–344. Also cited is Libonius's speech to young physicians, exhorting them to cultivate "love of man," to "share the pain" of the patient (p. 345).

19. Edmund D. Pellegrino and David C. Thomasma, "The Conflict between Autonomy and Beneficence," *Journal of Contemporary Health Law and Policy* 3 (1987): 23–46.

20. Edmund D. Pellegrino, "Moral Choice and the Good of the Patient: The Relationship of Duties, Rights, and Virtues," in *Proceedings of the Fourth Annual Arnold Schwartz Memorial Program* (New York: Arnold and Marie Schwartz College of Pharmacy and Health Sciences, Long Island University, 1983), pp. 44–68.

21. James F. Childress, *Who Should Decide? Paternalism in Health Care* (New York: Oxford University Press, 1982).

22. See the entire issue of *Theoretical Medicine* 5 (February 1984). Also Tom L. Beauchamp and James F. Childress, *Principles of Medical Ethics*, 4th ed. (New York: Oxford University Press, 1994), ch. 3, pp. 120–188; "Autonomy, Paternalism, Community," *Hastings Center Report* 14 (October 1984): 5–49.

23. Tom L. Beauchamp and Laurence B. McCullough, *Medical Ethics, the Responsibilities of Physicians* (Englewood Cliffs, N.J.: Prentice-Hall, 1984), ch. 2.

24. Pellegrino and Thomasma, *For the Patient's Good*, pp. 61–98.

25. Aristotle, *Nichomachean Ethics* 1137a 30, in *The Basic Works of Aritstotle*, ed. Richard McKeon (New York: Random House, 1941), p. 1019.

26. John Rawls, *A Theory of Justice* (Cambridge: Harvard University Press, 1971); Robert Nozick, *Anarchy, State, and Utopia* (New York: Basic Books, 1974).

27. The standard summary of the divisions of justice are borrowed from David Hollenbach, "Modern Catholic Teachings Concerning Justice," in *The Faith That Does Justice: Examining the Christian Sources of Social Change*, ed. John C. Haughey (New

York: Paulist Press, 1977), pp. 219–227. For a different and somewhat opposing view, see J. Brian Benestad, "The Catholic Concept of Social Justice: An Historical Perspective," *Communio* (Winter 1984): 364–381. Benestad argues that the current concepts of social justice in the United States are the result of a misunderstanding of Aquinas and Pius XI's writings. Benestad emphasizes the virtue of prudence and the duty of individuals to foster the common good, rather than rights and claims of individuals on society.

    28. See Owens, "Aristotelian Ethics."

    29. The essential points of his theory are summarized by John Rawls, *Theory of Justice*, pp. 302–303.

    30. Rawls, *Theory of Justice*, p. 62.

    31. Nozick, *Anarchy, State, and Utopia.*

    32. H. Tristram Engelhardt, Jr., "Shattuck Lecture: Allocating Scarce Medical Resources and the Availability of Organ Transplantation, Some Moral Presuppositions," *New England Journal of Medicine* 311 (July 5, 1984): 66–71.

9

Love and Justice in the Health Ministry: From Profession to Vocation—Theological Perspectives

> *A lamp to my feet is your word,*
> *A light to my path.*
> *I resolve and swear to keep*
> *Your just ordinances.*
> Psalm 119:105–106.

This final chapter develops the last steps of our argument about how love and justice would shape our vision of a just and loving health care ministry. We take up the argument in three sections, I) "The Theological Perspective," II) "Christocentric Health Care Ethics," and III) "The Call of the Whole Church to the Healing Ministry."

The religious person must attend to sources of moral guidance over and above philosophical analysis—to theological sources explicated in Scripture, tradition, and, for some, the teaching authority of the church. It is necessary to examine, first, Christian teaching on love and justice and their interrelationships, then how these Christian conceptions act as principles of discernment in health care and transform the obligations of philosophical ethics. When those obligations are seen as a "call" to a specific ministry, they become a genuine vocation—a call that cannot lightly be ignored.

THE THEOLOGICAL PERSPECTIVE

Love and justice are central to the whole of Christian theology. On this point, specifically Catholic Christian teachings are long, strong, and complex—far exceeding in richness any attempt to summarize them here.[1] Our focus will remain on the Christian tradition.

Christian notions of charity, *caritas* or *agapē*, derive their unique meaning from the life, teaching, and example of Jesus Christ. The central message of the Gospels is the announcement of the Good News of a God of love. He sent his only Son, who gave the ultimate demonstration of love when he suffered so that redemption might be made available to all mankind. Love of God and love of neighbor were Christ's daily exhortations to those who would follow him. The injunctions were not parallel but inclusive. Love of one another is the way to love God and find God's presence in human life. Love is therefore considered the touchstone to salvation, the only transforming power that can eradicate injustice from the world. Love is enjoined on all men and women because all are children of the same Father, who loves all persons.

Christian charity, epitomized in the gospel, went beyond the pagan notion of benevolence and beneficence, which itself could reach noble proportions on occasion.[2] Charity calls for love of all—enemy as well as friend, the unjust as well as the just. Christian charity, as St. Paul so eloquently expounded, calls for a higher degree of self-effacement than benevolence. The motive for doing good comes from the love of God.[3] Its highest expression calls for sacrifice even of one's own life. Without other-directed love, the natural virtues could become suspected of at least some taint of self-interest (e.g., the goals of a virtuous person to attain inner tranquility, etc.). To the extent that they are so tainted, they become less congruent with the perfection of human love that is charity.

The patristic tradition reinforced this gospel teaching by requiring charity because of the mutuality of obligation we owe each other since Christ is in every person.[4] It is Christ whom the Christian loves in self and others. The more perfect Christian charity is, the more it leads away from love of self and material goods and toward the dedication of self and material goods to the welfare of others. This is the ideal. It requires the kind of love that is free of utilitarian justification.

The differences between contemporary interpretations of beneficence and charity can be more concretely defined in health care ethics if we examine the spectrum of expressions possible for the principle of beneficence, philosophically construed. Thus, beneficence ranges from merely avoiding evil and/or harm to another (nonmaleficence) to doing good as long as it might not require inconvenience to the doer, to doing good at some inconvenience and risk to the doer, to doing good even at a great cost (altruism), and, finally, in its most heroic form, to sacrificing all one's goods or one's life for the other (heroism). Christian charity or agapeistic ethics calls for wishing and doing good precisely under those circumstances where it might be most difficult to justify doing so on rational grounds alone. Charity is, in some sense, "unreasonable" in that it violates philosophical standards of moderation. It becomes reasonable only when revelation counsels perfection and defines charitable action as other-directed specifically because that other is a person loved by God, even in the midst of his or her enmity toward the Christian.

The virtue of justice, like benevolence, is transformed, intensified, as Aquinas preferred to view it, by the Christian experience of grace. The pagan notion of justice, like that of contemporary theories, is ultimately practical and prudential. We owe others their due because we want them to give us our due and because we want to protect ourselves (enlightened self-interest) from the unjust claims of others. Justice contributes to the smooth running of society. Justice is a requirement for a peaceable society and the protection of legitimate self-interest. If we practice justice, we can assure happiness for all. Justice, in this view, is a claim we have on the community; compliance with the demands of justice is an obligation of communal living. In its highest expressions, it might be justified as owed to humans because they are worthy of respect and dignity.[5]

In the Christian view, however, justice has its deepest roots in love; it is an extension of the charity we should show to others. Not to do justice would be to relapse into self-interest, to turn from love of the other to love of self. Love, charity, *caritas*, *agapē*—each notion testifies that the claims of others upon us are the claims of brothers and sisters in Christ, loved equally by him and redeemed by God, and, by that fact, entitled to be loved.

In the Christian view, love generates and transmutes justice. As St. Augustine held, justice is the concern and love that Christians must show to others. Charity is for him "the root of all good."[6] It is truly the *vis a tergo* moving us to justice. Jesus dedicated his life to justice energized by a love that transcended the legalistic justice of the Pharisees at that time. In the Sermon on the Mount, Jesus calls his followers to live not only the letter but the spirit of the Law. His own life is the exemplification of the new justice. St. Paul repeats this exhortation when he calls upon Christians to "put on the new man."

In his own life, Jesus' concern, his practice of justice transmuted by charity, was for the poor, the sick, the troubled, the oppressed, and the outcast. He practiced justice transmuted by charity in concrete acts of beneficence toward specific persons. He did not argue for charity and justice in conformity with abstract principles. Christian justice does not focus on strict interpretations of what is owed in accordance with some calculus of claims and counterclaims. Instead, it offers the way of love illuminated by an ineffable guide. Christian justice does not obliterate the pagan virtue, but modulates and illuminates it by a principle of a very different sort, the principle of charity itself.[7] It is not knowledge that generates justice, as in Plato or Aristotle, but the loving concern of charity. Jesus on the cross asked the Father to forgive his crucifiers. He did not ask for the retributive justice of the Old Law.

The classical construals of justice in Plato, Aristotle, and the Roman Stoics intersect with the Christian notion and are worthy of continuing examination. The same is true of the intersections with contemporary ethics. Frankena, for example, suggests that the ethics of Christian charity is a theory of its own—"pure agapeism."[8] Justice philosophically derived and justice Christocentrically revealed cannot be fully equated. Their relationships and differences merit closer study in any attempt to answer whether, and how, Christian notions of love and justice modify the ethics of health care and its delivery today. Just how the natural and supernatural virtues complement, supplement, or transform each other is a subject of its own, too. One thing is certain, there will be consequences in the behaviors demanded by the modification of secular ethics. As Sokolowski avers: "It [the relation of natural and supernatural] has repercussions in Christian moral behavior, in education, and in the understanding Christians will have of their place in the world and in their social order."[9]

In the Christian view, justice is ultimately grounded in love—a charitable justice, i.e., rendering to others their due, in which "due" is not only what is legalistically owed but what is called for by love. Charity is the first principle of Christian justice. It could be similarly argued on philosophical grounds that justice is ultimately rooted in benevolence and beneficence. In this way, love can be the first principle of naturalistic and of Christian ethics.

Whether the Christian takes the Augustinian agapeistic, the Thomistic natural-law, or the religious existentialist perspective, one thing is undeniable—each Christian must respond personally to the life, way, and truth of Jesus Christ. The richness of that truth and its call to perfection are the wellsprings into which Christians must dip for inspiration and aspiration. This is not to expunge reason at all but to require that reason confront the unexpungeable reality of Christ's life and teaching. It is in this teaching that the intensification of the natural virtues is offered to the Christian through God's grace. Christ's healing becomes both the model and the obligation for practicing a special kind of love and justice in health care.

CHRISTOCENTRIC HEALTH CARE ETHICS: FROM PROFESSION TO VOCATION

The world today needs Christians who remain Christians.

Albert Camus, *Resistance, Rebellion, and Death.* [10]

Like all others, the Christian health professional is bound by the norms of philosophical medical ethics. From that source she derives principles, guidelines, rules, and codes that specify right from wrong actions, and, more important, the very criteria by which many such questions must be judged. For the Christian, this is not, however, the whole of ethics. To be sure, the Christian perspective does not add another whole set of specific prescriptions; but the Christian ethic enjoins one overriding principle: love of God and neighbor.

The distinguishing factor of Christocentric ethics is the fact of revelation—a point that Frankena acknowledged in his classification of Christian ethics as agapeistic. [11] This difference does not yield precise indications, rules, or guidelines to determine what should be done in every given situation. Nor does it, of necessity, preclude the use of deontological or utilitarian principles in this or that decision. It requires only that any principle or ethical theory conform to the spirit of love and justice exemplified in the life, work, and teaching of Jesus Christ.

The Christian perspective, therefore, provides principles of discernment more than a code of rules for action. What it lacks in specificity it gains in insight. It is a beacon and a compass that individual

Christians and the Church must use to find the direction that their faith requires them to follow. This is a task at once more demanding and perilous. The call is to perfection—and the precise recipe for success is not available. Further, as times change and as new technological advances appear, the answer must continuously be reexamined and retested.

Christocentric ethics is, therefore, in its deepest sense, "beyond" ethics. Romano Guardini puts it very well: "Once we restrict the word ethics to its modern specific sense of moral principles, it no longer accurately covers the Sermon on the Mount. What Jesus revealed there on the mountainside was no mere ethical code, but a whole new existence."[12] This is not to dispose of ethics or law. Law impels us to limit self-interest for fear of punishment and thus assures an orderly society based on rights. Ethics impels us to limit self interest as rational beings who recognize duties to others, and it thus assures a concerned and responsible social life. Religion impels us to limit self-interest because God asks us to do so out of love for him and his creatures, and it thus assures a caring society. This is something of what Guardini means when he says: "Only in love is genuine fulfillment of the ethical possible."[13]

Philosophical ethics can define the proper relationship between human beings but not between God and humans or between humans as God wants those relationships to be. As Sokolowski comments on the relation between the natural and the supernatural: "It is not enough to continue inspecting the two terms of the distinction, the natural and the graced, in an effort to find what is common and what is differing in them. It is necessary to move to different ground and to pay attention to the distinction itself, not just to its terms."[14]

What he means by "paying attention to the distinction itself" is what he calls a theology of disclosure, a new way of looking at old realities, of seeing that what is need not be that way.[15] A Christocentric ethic, therefore, does not repudiate philosophical ethics but transvalues its highest principles, justice and beneficence, into love and thereby carries them beyond the highest human aspirations.

There are, of course, specific moral principles and rules to guide individual religions. Catholics, for example, are guided by the promulgations of the Moral Code for Catholic Hospitals, the pastoral letters of the bishops, the writings of the theologians, and the teachings of the popes and the official magisterium. But these sources are, all in their own ways, the products of discernment—of the way any institutional church "reads" Christ's call to love and justice in health care. There are numerous instances today in which such principles of discernment are needed to guide specific decisions and actions. These touch on some of the most important issues in health care today. Let us turn now to a brief examination of some selected aspects of contemporary health care ethics to see where the vectors of Christian discernment point.

In the changed sociopolitical, economic, and scientific climate within which medicine is practiced today, there are conflicting conceptions of the healing relationship. Earlier in this book we attempted a phenomenological analysis of the healing relationship. Some of the formulations of this relationship would be more congenial to a Christian perspective than others. Thus, it would not require a high degree of Christian discernment to discern that a biological model of the physician-patient or healing relationship would be insufficient, if not antithetic to a Christian interpretation of healing or helping. The same could be said of the relationship viewed as a legal contract or a commodity relationship, or as strongly paternalistic. Other models—covenant, friendship, or fidelity to promise—would be more congruent.[16]

All the models cited have some verisimilitude. Without denying this fact, it is what the model perceives as primary that is of utmost importance. Thus, strong paternalism would rarely, if ever, be countenanced, while weak paternalism could be.[17] A strictly libertarian relationship would not be consistent, since it would forbid intervention in suicide or euthanasia, for example. With these exceptions, respect for the autonomy of the competent patient as a human person would not only be consistent but required. So, too, would respect for the respective agency of patient and physician, with neither imposing on the other except where grave harm was in prospect. Neither could ask the other to act contrary to conscience.

Likewise, a strictly contractual model of the healing relationship is insufficient from a Christian perspective. The contractual model requires only a minimalistic ethic—one that obligates the patient and the physician to fulfill the terms of an agreement and nothing more. This model calls for the minimal amount of beneficence. Rather, it is contrived to reduce dependence upon either the physician's benevolence or his fidelity to promises. It is precisely those features of the relationship that a contract cannot cover—the uncertainties inherent in the clinical situation and reliance on the fidelity and goodwill of the physician and patient—that charity most clearly regulates.

The most distinctive characteristic of a healing relationship motivated by the Christian perspective is the higher degree of self-effacement it requires as a matter of course. Even on strictly philosophical grounds, the vulnerability of the sick person imposes a special responsibility not to take advantage of the patient. In a more positive sense, the physician commits himself to some degree of suppression of his own self-interest, comfort, and preferences in order to serve his patient. This is the "higher devotion" that should motivate the medical profession.[18]

From the Christian perspective, self-effacement is an obligation of charity toward others, motivated by love and without the motive of self-interest. Being imperfect, few physicians are expected to practice heroic levels of self-sacrifice. But a Christian physician has a moral obligation to be compassionate, considerate, and courteous even to her "difficult" patients, to be available to them even at some considerable inconvenience to herself, and to be solicitous for their needs. The Christian perspective precludes some of the excessive expressions of self-pity we see today on the part of physicians, the complaints about income, work hours, delayed gratification, or the justification for recreation at the expense of commitment to patient needs. It precludes also the attitude of some physicians who feel that, having worked so hard and paid so much for a medical education, they are entitled to "get it back" financially, or in prestige, privileges, and prerogatives.

Self-effacement, it must be said, however binding it may be in naturalistic and Christocentric medical ethics, does not require neglect of one's personal or familial well-being. Physicians are entitled to develop and grow as persons, to enjoy recreation, to serve their families, and to provide for their own material needs. Extreme interpretations of the obligation to self-effacement can be as morally unsound as its neglect. Indeed, immoderate self-sacrifice is too often an excuse for an inability to balance conflicting obligations or even for deliberately neglecting some of them.

The issue is really one of balance—knowing when legitimate self-interest should dominate and when self-effacement is the product of constant reflection and emotional maturity—something for which no instant formula is at hand. Suffice it to say that prudence, the virtue St. Thomas thought so central to the Christian life, is the virtue to be cultivated here.[19]

The charitable self-effacement implicit in a Christian vocation to the health ministry leads the physician away from a series of activities at the moral margin—things neither illegal nor contravened by professional codes but nonetheless fraught with compromises of Christian conceptions of charity and justice. We refer here to most of the practices associated with today's commercialistic, competitive, and entrepreneurial medicine, e.g., investing in the health care "industry," owning shares in hospitals and nursing homes, patenting medical procedures, and working in for-profit or corporately owned hospitals, clinics, and HMOs. The list of investment "opportunities" in health care open to physicians grows daily. The profit motive sooner or later must conflict with the deference owed the sick person by virtue of the inequality of a relationship in which one of the parties is ill and dependent upon the other. Making a profit from the sickness of others in order to produce a return to investors comes too close to exploitation, even in the best circumstances.

The ethics of business, as it is presently understood, cannot be relied upon to guarantee that extra measure of solicitude that Christian ministry to the sick requires. The Christian physician has a positive responsibility to resist, and even to refuse, to participate in actions that endanger a patient out of motives of fiscal necessity. The "economic transfer," for example, of the patient whose insurance is insufficient to pay for care in a private institution is a growing example in point that is causing ethical dilemmas for conscientious physicians.

Equally to be condemned is the practice, becoming too frequent these days, of physicians' asking whether the patient is insured adequately before seeing him. In the same vein, excessive fees, overutilization of diagnostic or therapeutic services, exuberant advertising, maneuvers to dominate the market, and a whole host of morally marginal business practices would be eschewed by any physician who claimed Christian authenticity for this ministry to the sick. The physician's "right" to treat whom he pleases would, in a Christian view of medical ethics, be limited.

Another form of behavior antithetical to the Christian notion of love and justice is the refusal to treat certain kinds of patients who represent a threat to the physician. We refer here especially to AIDS patients. Instances are increasing of physicians, nurses, and other health professionals who avoid caring for these patients. Some even take the view that AIDS patients are victims of their own self-abuse and not worthy of care. Similar attitudes are evident with respect to alcoholics, smokers, the very obese, or diabetics who do not follow their dietary regimens.

In short, a Christian vocation of healing imposes a standard of commutative justice weighted heavily in the direction of benevolence and beneficence, even at the expense of inconvenience, cost, and some danger to the physician. Simple nonmaleficence would not suffice. Such an interpretation of beneficence is, of course, not closed to the non-Christian. It is often exhibited by those without the Christian imperative, to the scandal of Christian physicians. But for the Christian, such behavior is a matter of moral obligation. The Christian physician or health professional cannot live a life of contradiction in which professional and personal morality are divorced. Such a state is inconsistent with even the most rudimentary interpretations of authentic Christian living, to say nothing of a Christian vocation.

In the realms of distributive and social justice, a Christocentric ethic would, of necessity, favor some interpretations of justice over others. Thus, Nozick's fundamental principle of protecting the inequalities of the natural lottery would be the antithesis of a Christian perspective. The Christian vocation is quite specifically oriented to a charitable redress of the inequities of nature or circumstance. It is, in fact, precisely to the losers in the natural lottery—the sick, the poor, the outcast—that Christ addressed his personal ministry and his Sermon on the Mount. This is the basis for the preferential option for the poor that inspires the best Christian institutions. [20]

Likewise, the distribution of goods and rationing on principles of social worth, merit, productivity, ability to pay, age, or burden on society would be hard to justify. Egalitarian principles of justice, like Rawls's, would have much more claim on the Christian, though not for the reason Rawls adduces—that is to say, not because we ourselves might be the disadvantaged persons. Rather, the Christian should show love and justice to all equally, because all are our brothers and sisters under God, not because we might need help ourselves some day.

As promised at the start of the last chapter, two kinds of justice we did not treat earlier require mention at this point: retributive and compensatory justice. Retributive justice treats of the redress of injury by punishment of the wrongdoer. In health care it is expressed today as an option to control costs by limiting care to those who are responsible for their ill-health—the smoker, the overeater, the victim of venereal disease, and the drug addict. An even sterner view of justice would interpret withholding care as just punishment for past indiscretions. This form of justice goes counter to a Christocentric health care ministry as we have defined it here.

Compensatory justice makes amends for injustices in the past. In health care, it would call for extra solicitude for the poor, for minorities, for those who have not had access to health care, and for those badly treated by the natural lottery. It is applicable, too, in admission criteria to medical schools and such things as faculty and hospital appointments. In the Christian view, compensatory justice is an obligation implicit in the call to perfection. A preferential option for the poor, the disadvantaged, and all who have been ill favored by history, environment, heredity, or political or social circumstance is a necessary extrapolation of the virtue of Christian charity.

In the realm of social justice, the Christian vocation to health care would impose an obligation to participate in designing and operating institutions and policies that would result in a just and equitable distribution of health care as well as other socially important services. Personal involvement is required of the individual health professional, of the health professions as corporate entities, and of the entire Christian community. The provision of just and merciful health care to all is thus a shared responsibility of all Christians in social justice. Advocacy for the sick, in all its dimensions, is a responsibility, especially today, when our social mores tend to accept inequality and two-level medical care as justifiable.

These implications of the Christian concept of social justice are not widely acknowledged by Catholics or other Christians. Too many widely "delegate" their own responsibility to health professionals, health care institutions, or governmental or voluntary agencies. All Christians share a mutual responsibility to assure that health care institutions—Catholic, Christian, or secular—do in fact act with justice and love. As members of democratic societies, we are expected to use the means available in those societies to shape our institutions. Those who are bureaucrats have a special Christian vocation to work within their institutional contexts to see that those institutions perform in morally justifiable ways.

Distributive and social justice are also obligations of the institutional Church. Since Christ provided so many examples of his solicitude for the sick, the healing ministry is an essential part of the evangelical ministry of the whole Church. Pope John Paul II has only recently reaffirmed the importance of that ministry. He reaffirms the

Good Samaritan parable as a model for Christians, who should be impelled by love and justice to help the sufferings of the sick.[21]

The institutional Church must, as it has for centuries, remain involved in sponsoring health care institutions today for several very good reasons. First, hospitals and health care institutions, as we know them today, were born under the aegis of the Church. The reasons for them are as cogent today as they were then. Second, the Church-sponsored institution is increasingly the last resort of the poor in a community and the only safety net available. Third, the religious hospital is the only place in which religious medical moral principles can be exemplified and applied daily in medical decisions. This option in medical models must be available to anyone so committed. Fourth, hospital and health care agencies provide concrete examples of what being a Christian means. To be a Christian is to infuse everything we do with the message of love and justice Christ gave to us, a message that forever changes the way we are expected to live with each other.

THE CALL OF THE WHOLE CHURCH TO THE HEALING MINISTRY

It is important to reassert the vocation, the call, of the whole Church to the imitation of Christ. Today, for example, Catholic hospitals everywhere are tempted by fiscal exigencies to retreat from the care of the poor, to sell out to for-profit corporations, or to compromise with the commercialization and "monetarizing" practices adopted by their "competitors." Yet it is precisely the ubiquity and the noncompassionate nature of many of today's fiscal exigencies that impose an ever greater necessity for continued involvement of the institutional Church. Healing has always been essential to the Church's evangelical mission and is also witness to the world that Christian belief makes a difference in the way Christians live.

We have argued elsewhere, but will not repeat the argument here, that Catholic hospitals and health care institutions can "compete" in today's health care milieu without the compromise of moral integrity and that they must do so to remain faithful to the call we all share to care for the sick.[22] Survival, so much discussed by Catholic professionals and boards, cannot be at the expense of compromise or capitulation. This means a degree of cooperation, a concrete practice of charity, among Catholic and Christian hospitals not yet fully tried. It means greater personal and financial support by Christian laypeople and greater volunteer assistance on a scale not yet practiced.

Catholics and Christians have an additional obligation to all of society. By uniting in the care of the sick, the poor, and the dependent members of a society, they demonstrate the need for love in any society. This is a message easy to repudiate when preached in the abstract, but difficult to ignore when witnessed in action. It is a message vital to today's world, where every force seems to favor divisiveness. Communities cannot survive without something they love in common, some things that transcend the uninhibited self-interest of the competitive spirit.

All Christians have a vocation—that is, a call from God to follow Christ, "to proclaim the exploits of God who called us, out of darkness into this marvelous light."[23] Within that larger call, each person is also called to follow Christ in some specific activity. Whatever that activity may be—exalted or humble—it becomes illuminated by the light of faith and love. "Everyone has his own vocation in which he has been called; let him keep to it."[24]

A vocation is a grace, the stirring of the mind and the will which can be accepted or rejected. When it is accepted consciously, an activity becomes a Christian vocation. In the case of the health worker, the conscious response to God's call transmutes a profession into a vocation.

A vocation differs from a profession. A profession is a self-generated declaration of dedication to a certain standard of ethical behavior. A vocation is the same kind of declaration, but one that has its source in a call from God and a desire to do God's will, to be a witness of the gospel message through a specific life activity.

For the Christian health professional—doctor, nurse, dentist, or other health worker—it is not sufficient to remain faithful to the moral imperatives of a philosophical or naturalistic ethic. A Christian vocation includes the obligations assumed by other professionals, but they must be supplemented, enriched, and made congruent with the spirit of a justice transmuted by love that flows from a Christocentric ethic. In a vocation, the seminal principles of beneficence and justice, central to philosophical ethics, are interpreted in the light of the spirit of the Scripture through the tradition of the Church and the special teachings of the official magisterium.

The objection will be raised that all we have argued is unrealistic and far from the behavior of physicians or hospitals. The allegation is often made that not-for-profit hospitals, Christian and non-Christian, do make a profit, too, and that the physician's fee is also a form of profit. Why, then, should we be so self-righteous about for-profit hospitals or the commercial aspect of medical practices? Have not physicians been the staunchest supporters of the free-enterprise system, of untrammeled and unregulated practice, of free choice for patients? Are they not the major opponents of nationalized or socialized centrally planned systems and fee schedules, etc.?

Much of this is true. Indeed, we would go further and say that many physicians and their professional organizations are seeing today the local extrapolations of economic and political philosophies they themselves espoused. Now it turns out that those philosophies are hurtful to them and to their patients. For some, they are simply the fulfillment of their hopes for medicine as a free-market enterprise. Like the automotive industry, we are for competition until it hurts us.

While some of this is true, some is not. Not-for-profit hospitals do not make profit the same way that for-profit hospitals do. For one thing, their "excess of revenue over expenditures" does not go into the pockets of the hospital trustees or distant investors. It all goes into capital improvement or expansion for other activities related to the improvement of patient care. This is very different from the primary orientation of a corporation entity to provide a return to investors. That return is a moral obligation, too. It is the way that the obligation to maximize the investor's money and the obligation to the sick conflict that constitutes the major objection to for-profit medicine.

Fees do contain some excess of revenue over expenditure. Presumably, that is the charge for the physician's time and effort—what he receives after he has paid his expenses of practice. The question morally is not whether he should be paid for his time and effort but how much is legitimate. There is no doubt that many fees are not morally defensible and some investments are morally unconscionable.

CONCLUSION

Admitting all of this does not vitiate the arguments of this book. It is in the nature of ethical discourse to define what ought to be done—not justify what is, in fact, done. The present or past activities of physicians or the profession as a whole, of hospitals, religious or not, are not self-justifying. What we tried to do is derive what are morally defensible norms—what *should be*, rather than *what is*.

Ultimately the Christian healing ministry rests on the mystery of the patient who was Christ, whose suffering and victory was a redemption for the whole human race. Pope Paul VI, commenting on this mystery, constructed a vision of the healing ministry that fuses the idea of the profession indissolubly with the idea of a vocation.[25] His call is one to which each Christian health professional must respond in the measure God's grace and his other capabilities allow. It is a vision that the committed Christian will grasp—without the laborious argumentation we have provided here.

NOTES

1. See John Langan, "What Jerusalem Says to Athens"; David Hollenbach, "Modern Catholic Teachings Concerning Justice"; and William J. Walsh and John P. Langan, "Patristic Social Consciousness: The Church and the Poor," in *The Faith That Does Justice: Examining the Christian Sources of Social Change*, ed. John C. Haughey (New York: Paulist Press, 1977), pp. 152–180, 234–263, and 113–151, respectively.

2. See Marcus Tullius Cicero, *De officiis*, trans. Walter Miller (Cambridge: Harvard University Press, 1968), the *vade mecum* of later Stoic morality.

3. For an exposition of Paul's notion of love and justice, see John C. Haughey, "Jesus and the Justice of God," in *The Faith That Does Justice*, ed. Haughey pp. 282–288.

4. Walsh and Langan, "Patristic Social Consciousness."

5. David C. Thomasma, "The Basis of Medicine and Religion: Respect for Persons," *Hospital Progress* 60 (September 1979): 54–57, 90.

6. St. Augustine, *Sermon 72*, 4 as cited in Walsh and Langan, "Patristic Social Consciousness," n. 18, p. 118.

7. The question of the continuity or discontinuity of the supernatural and the natural virtues is still an intriguing one. Robert Sokolowski has examined this relationship in a brilliant monograph, *The God of Faith and Reason* (Notre Dame, Ind.: University of Notre Dame Press, 1982).

8. William Frankena, *Ethics*, 2d ed. (Englewood Cliffs, N.J.: Prentice-Hall, 1973).

9. Robert Sokolowski, *God of Faith and Reason*, p. xi.

10. Albert Camus, *Resistance, Rebellion, and Death*, trans. Justin O'Brien (New York: Alfred Knopf, 1961), p. 70.

11. Frankena, *Ethics*.

12. Romano Guardini, *The Lord* (Chicago: Henry Regnery, 1954), p. 79.

13. Guardini, *The Lord,* p. 84.

14. Sokolowski, *God of Faith and Reason,* p. 90.

15. Sokolowski, *God of Faith and Reason,* pp. 90–103.

16. See William F. May, *The Physician's Covenant* (Philadelphia: Westminster Press, 1983); Pedro Lain Entralgo, *La relacion medico-enfermo: historia y teoria* (Madrid: Revista de Occidente, 1964), pp. 235–288; and Edmund D. Pellegrino, "Toward a Reconstruction of Medical Morality: The Primacy of the Act of Profession and the Fact of Illness," *Journal of Medicine and Philosophy* 4, no. 1 (1979): 32–56.

17. See the discussion of strong and weak paternalism in James F. Childress, *Who Should Decide? Paternalism in Health Care* (New York: Oxford University Press, 1982), pp. 102–112.

18. Harvey Cushing, "The Common Devotion," in *Consecratio Medici and Other Papers* (Boston: Little Brown, 1929), pp. 3–13.

19. Josef Pieper, *The Four Cardinal Virtues* (Notre Dame, Ind.: University of Notre Dame Press, 1966); also St. Thomas Aquinas, *Summa Theologiae,* vol. 36, trans. Thomas Gilby (New York: McGraw-Hill/Blackfriars, 1974), II–II, art. 47, responses 4–5, pp. 14–21.

20. See Laurence J. O'Connell, "The Preferential Option for the Poor and Health Care in the U.S.," in *Medical Ethics: A Guide for Health Professionals,* ed. John F. Monagle and David C. Thomasma (Frederick, Md.: Aspen, 1988).

21. Pope John Paul II, *Salvifici Doloris* (Washington, D.C.: United States Catholic Conference, 1984).

22. Edmund D. Pellegrino, "Catholic Hospitals: Survival without Moral Compromise," *Health Progress* 66, no. 4 (1985): 42–49.

23. 1 Peter 2:9. See the entry "Vocation," in *A Catholic Dictionary,* 3d ed., ed. Donald Attwater (New York: Macmillan, 1958), p. 520.

24. 1 Cor. 7:20. Also "Vocation," in *A Catholic Dictionary,* ed. Attwater.

25. Pope Paul VI, "*Allocution a Des medecins*" in *Documents Pontificaux de Paul VI* (St. Maurice, Switzerland: Editions Saint Augustin, 1969), p. 701.

Subject Index

Name Index

Adams, John 57
Adkins, Janet 79
American Medical Association 86
Amundsen, Darrel 51
Anderson, Douglas 11
Anthony, E. James 52, 125
St. Thomas Aquinas 1, 40, 76, 82, 125, 161
Aristotle 1, 144
St. Augustine of Hippo 13, 56, 65, 142, 160

Baby Doe 89
Baby Fae 89
Ba-Sela, Ariel 144
Beauchamp, Tom L. 144
Benestad, J. Brian 145
Benner, Patricia 28, 37
Bennett, John C. 40, 51
Bergsma, Jurrit 25, 52
Bernardin, Joseph Cardinal 41, 51, 66
Bleich, J. David 104
Elizabeth Bouvia 89
Buddha 75
Burns, Chester 144
Byrd, Randolph C. 51

Caldwell, Alethea O. 124
Callahan, Daniel 66
Calvin, John 43
Camus, Albert 36, 38, 82, 84, 103, 160
Caplan, Arthur L. 25, 143
Carse, James P. 11

Cassell, Eric 14, 16, 25, 52, 125
Catholic Health Association of the United States 124
Childress, James F. 144, 161
Cicero 160
Cousins, Norman 25
Cruzan, Nancy 44, 89
Curran, Charles E. 143
Cushing, Harvey 33, 38, 103, 161

Dawkins, Richard 65
Descartes, René 80
Dewey, John 5, 11
Diamond, Eugene 52
Dodd, Charles H. 125
Donahue, John R. 143

Edelstein, Ludwig 37, 103
Egan, Timothy 83
Engel, Gerard L. 37
Engelhardt, H. Tristram, Jr. 65, 74–75, 77, 82, 117, 143, 145
Entralgo, Pedro Lain 161

Father Damien 97
Finkelstein, Katherine Eban 123
Foulkes, Siegmund H. 47, 52, 125
Fourth Council of the Lateran 42
St. Francis 97
Frank, Peter 94
Frankena, William 67, 82, 149, 160
Frankl, Viktor 46, 52

166

Printed in the United States
88511LV00008B/76/A